Fighting Cancer

with Vitamins and Antioxidants

Kedar N. Prasad, Ph.D.,
and
K. Che Prasad, M.S., M.D.

Healing Arts Press
Rochester, Vermont • Toronto, Canada

Healing Arts Press
One Park Street
Rochester, Vermont 05767
www.HealingArtsPress.com

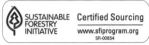

Text stock is SFI certified

Healing Arts Press is a division of Inner Traditions International

First edition originally published in 1984 by Nutrition Publishing House under the title
Vitamins Against Cancer
Second edition published in 1989 by Healing Arts Press
Third edition published in 1994 by Healing Arts Press under the title *Vitamins in Cancer Prevention and Treatment*
Fourth edition published in 2001 by Healing Arts Press under the title *Fight Cancer with Vitamins and Supplements*
Fifth edition published in 2011 by Healing Arts Press under the title *Fighting Cancer with Vitamins and Antioxidants*

Note to the reader: Although every effort was made to provide current reliable information based on scientific data, the authors and publishers accept no liability for any errors or omissions that may be present in this book, and no liability is accepted arising directly or indirectly as a result of reading of any part or from any other use of this book. The readers should consult their physicians or other health practitioners before adopting any recommendation presented in this book.

Library of Congress Cataloging-in-Publication Data
Prasad, Kedar N.
  Fighting cancer with vitamins and antioxidants / Kedar N. Prasad and K. Che Prasad.
    p. cm.
  Summary: "The most up-to-date and complete resource on the powerful benefits of micronutrients for cancer treatment and prevention" — Provided by publisher.
  Rev. ed. of: Fight cancer with vitamins and supplements. 2001.
  Includes bibliographical references and index.
  ISBN 978-1-59477-423-2 (pbk.) — ISBN 978-1-59477-807-0 (e-book)
  1. Cancer—Diet therapy. 2. Vitamin therapy. 3. Dietary supplements. 4. Cancer—Chemoprevention. I. Prasad, Che. II. Prasad, Kedar N. Fight cancer with vitamins and supplements. III. Title.
  RC271.V58P73 2011
  616.99'40654—dc23
                                                                        2011035147

Printed and bound in the United States by Lake Book Manufacturing
The text stock is SFI certified. The Sustainable Forestry Initiative® program promotes sustainable forest management.

10 9 8 7 6 5 4 3 2 1

Text design and layout by Virginia Scott Bowman
This book was typeset in Garamond Premier Pro and Myriad Pro with Helvetica, Gill Sans, and Myriad Pro used as display typefaces

To send correspondence to the authors of this book, mail a first-class letter to the authors c/o Inner Traditions • Bear & Company, One Park Street, Rochester, VT 05767, and we will forward the communication.

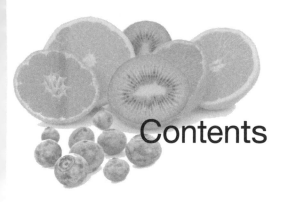

Contents

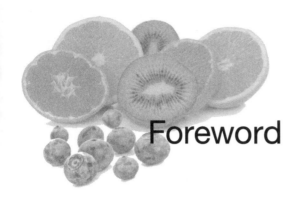

Foreword

Much has been achieved during the past fifty years in relation to the prevention and early detection of several cancers. For example, most lung cancers would not occur if nobody smoked, and many early and therefore curable breast cancers can now be detected by mammography, or early and eminently curable large-bowel cancers detected by colonoscopy. Similarly, advances in cancer treatment have resulted in the prolonged survival or even the cure of many whose outlook was previously regarded as poor.

In spite of all this progress there are still many hurdles to jump in the successful prevention and treatment of many cancers. This is where *Fighting Cancer with Vitamins and Antioxidants* comes into the picture. The authors, a father-son duo of published scientists, lucidly describe the evidence and potential value of vitamins and several other micronutrient supplements in both the prevention and treatment of cancer.

A major feature of this book is the clarity with which complex concepts, such as the immune system, antioxidants, free radicals, how supplements work, and carcinogens in our environment, lifestyle, and diet are explained. These concepts and terms are often quoted in popular literature without explanation, leaving many, especially lay readers, in the dark.

Important to the authors' approach is a reliance on scientific data and rational evidence. They emphasize the major distinction between the preventive and therapeutic approach to micronutrient use. They also believe that micronutrient supplements, used alone, are not a cure-all or panacea, but rather adjuncts to other strategies, such as diet in cancer prevention, and surgery, radiotherapy, or chemotherapy in cancer treatment. The misuse and risks of inappropriate micronutrient use are outlined in the book. The authors stress using supplements in conjunction with the advice of a physician or other relevant health professional, a policy I strongly support.

In cancer prevention, the authors propose a strategy that combines the avoidance of exposure to environmental carcinogens such as smoking with a healthy diet and lifestyle changes including regular exercise and the daily use of multiple micronutrients, the nature and dosage of which is based on currently available data.

Author Kedar N. Prasad is also an expert and published radio-biologist. Because of this expertise he has included an interesting and novel section on cancer risk after diagnostic doses of radiation, a relatively poorly researched field, especially when it comes to cancer prevention. In cancer prevention of this group of people, the authors propose the addition of antioxidants to currently practiced strategies of radiation dose reduction. The authors also mention the potential value of antioxidant use among other groups exposed to various forms of radiation, such as pilots, airline stewards, radiation and radiology workers, and even those who use cell phones heavily. Clearly, further research is needed.

The place of micronutrient supplements as an adjunct to radiation, chemotherapy, or experimental treatments such as hyperthermia is the subject of controversy. Many oncologists and physicians believe that antioxidants and perhaps other supplements protect normal cells as well as cancer cells from radiation damage, thereby making such cancer treatment less effective than expected. The authors of this book, however, argue that there is sufficient scientific evidence to show that an appropriately dosed combination of multiple supplements protects normal body cells but not cancer cells, thereby decreasing the adverse side effects of radiation and possibly of chemotherapy. Important clinical research is needed to resolve this controversy, and the authors quite correctly suggest the conducting of well-designed intervention studies with the use of appropriately dosed multiple supplements.

This book is clearly written and based on science and current data. It provides a stimulus for much-needed research in some unresolved areas of cancer prevention and cancer treatment. The book is an important contribution to the prevention and treatment of human cancers, and the role that micronutrient supplements play within it.

GABRIEL KUNE, M.D.,
EMERITUS PROFESSOR OF SURGERY,
THE UNIVERSITY OF MELBOURNE,
AUSTRALIA

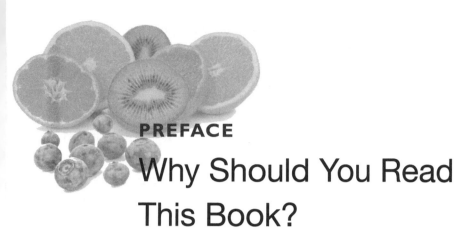

Why Should You Read This Book?

Despite extensive research on the role of diet, lifestyle, and antioxidants in cancer prevention, the incidence of cancer in the United States has increased from 1.2 million new cases per year only a decade ago to about 1.5 million cases per year in 2009. The current recommendation of consuming a diet rich in antioxidants, low in fat, and high in fiber, although very rational, has not had significant impact on reducing the incidence of cancer. Increased oxidative stress from the production of excessive amounts of free radicals, along with the effects of chronic inflammation, plays a major role in the initiation and progression of cancer.

Micronutrients, especially antioxidants, have been shown to help ameliorate these effects; therefore, they have great potential for reducing the risk of cancer. Unfortunately, some clinical studies in which a single antioxidant was used in populations at high risk for developing cancer (such as heavy tobacco smokers), revealed an increased cancer risk in the antioxidant-treated group. These results have called into question the potential value of antioxidants in cancer prevention. This revised edition of *Fighting Cancer with Vitamins and Antioxidants* discusses the questions that have arisen from these studies and proposes solutions. The solutions include changes to the diet and lifestyle together with daily supplementation with a specific multiple-micronutrient preparation containing dietary and endogenous (made by the body) antioxidants for reducing the risk of cancer.

The U.S. mortality rate from cancer has not changed significantly during the past several decades, in spite of extensive research and the development of new treatment methods and drugs. The American Cancer Society estimates that in 1950 the death rate from cancer was about 194 per 100,000. In 2006 this value was 180.7 per 100,000. The effectiveness of standard cancer treatment, which includes radiation therapy, chemotherapy, and surgery, has reached a plateau for many solid tumors. In addition, damage to normal tissue occurs during radiation and chemotherapy. While some therapies have been successful—reducing the risk of recurrence of breast cancer with tamoxifen, for example—there are often no effective strategies to reduce the risk of recurrence of the other primary tumors or the development of second cancers among cancer survivors. There are also no effective strategies to prolong the survival time of patients who have become unresponsive to all therapies. Supplementation with a multiple-micronutrient preparation has great potential to enhance the effectiveness of standard therapy, reduce the risk of recurrence of primary tumors, reduce the risk of developing new cancer among survivors, and increase survival time.

However, the role of antioxidants in cancer therapy has become controversial, and many oncologists discourage patients from taking antioxidants before or after therapy. This revised edition of *Fighting Cancer with Vitamins and Antioxidants* discusses the reasons behind these controversies and proposes a specific preparation of multiple micronutrients, including antioxidants, for those receiving standard therapy, those in remission, and those who have become unresponsive to all therapies.

Recent studies suggest an increased risk of cancer among individuals who receive diagnostic doses of radiation (such as during mammograms, CT scans, chest X-rays, dental X-rays, and nuclear medicine procedures), radiation workers (individuals working with X-ray equipment and employees at nuclear power plants), and frequent fliers (pilots and crews of aircraft). The revised edition of *Fighting Cancer with Vitamins and Antioxidants* discusses in detail the cancer risk among these groups and suggests a specific multiple-micronutrient preparation to reduce the risk of cancer among them. The recommendations should be adopted only in consultation with a physician.

KEDAR N. PRASAD, PH.D.
K. CHE PRASAD, M.S., M.D.

1 Common Misconceptions about Cancer

During the past three decades, extensive research on antioxidants, diet, and cancer prevention and treatment has been published in peer-reviewed journals and gives an inconsistent message to the public and health professionals regarding the value of antioxidants. Many popular magazines and books have also reported contradicting claims regarding the usefulness of antioxidants for maintaining good health and preventing or treating cancer.

Micronutrients include antioxidants, B vitamins, and certain minerals such as iron, copper, manganese, selenium, and zinc. Some antioxidants are made in the body, such as glutathione, alpha-lipoic acid, coenzyme Q10, and antioxidant enzyme. We will refer to them as endogenous antioxidants. Other antioxidants are found in the diet, such as vitamin A, beta-carotene, vitamin E, and vitamin C. We will refer to them as dietary antioxidants. Both endogenous and dietary antioxidants are absolutely essential for our growth and survival. In addition, antioxidants protect our bodies against damage caused by free radicals. Free radicals are atoms, molecules, or ions with unpaired electrons that are formed as by-products whenever oxygen is used by cells. Free radicals can be derived from oxygen or nitrogen and are symbolized by a dot: •.

Small amounts of free radicals play an important role in several biochemical reactions and in the stability of genetic activity that is necessary for our survival. Excessive amounts of free radicals can damage all parts of the cells, including genetic material. They play a central role in initiation and progression of human cancer. In 1900 the first organic free radical, triphenylmethyl radical, was identified by Moses Gomberg of the University of Michigan in the United States.

Although most nutrition scientists agree with the idea that changes in the diet and lifestyle may reduce the risk of cancer, the value of micronutrients, including antioxidants, in cancer prevention or treatment remains controversial and the subject of extensive debate. As a result, a number of misconceptions concerning the value of supplementary micronutrients exist among the general public and many health professionals. In an effort to reduce confusion, some of them are discussed herein.

Misconception 1: The more supplementary micronutrients, including antioxidants, you take, the better you will feel.

Fact: This belief can be dangerous to your health. Consumption of excessive amounts of certain micronutrients may cause severe damage to your body. For instance, taking large amounts of vitamin A (25,000 IU or more per day over a long period of time) may lead to liver and skin toxicity. Vitamin A, even at lower doses of 10,000 IU or more, can increase the risk of birth defects in pregnant women and of bone fractures in older women. Excessive intake of selenium—400 micrograms (mcg) or more per day over a long period of time—may cause cataracts (an eye disease in which the lens becomes opaque). Taking vitamin B_6 (50 mg or more per day over a long period of time) can induce peripheral neuropathy (numbness in the extremities), which is reversible upon discontinuation of the vitamin.

Misconception 2: All the different forms of vitamins C and E have similar effects on cancer cells and normal cells.

Fact: This statement has been proved untrue in many experiments. For example, vitamin E in the form of d-alpha-tocopheryl succinate is more potent than other forms, such as d-alpha-tocopherol, d-alpha-tocopheryl acetate, or d-alpha-tocopheryl nicotinate, in curtailing the growth of cancer cells, but it has no effect on normal cells. Vitamin C is sold commercially as ascorbic acid, sodium ascorbate, or calcium ascorbate. Ascorbic acid at high doses can cause upset stomach in some people. Sodium ascorbate at high doses can increase the concentration of sodium in the urine, which has been shown to increase the risk of chemically induced bladder cancer in animals. Calcium ascorbate appears to be the most suitable form of vitamin C for reducing the growth of cancer cells without affecting the growth of normal cells.

Misconception 3: The addition of trace minerals, such as iron, copper, and manganese to many multiple-vitamin preparations containing vitamin C is good for your health.

Fact: Your body needs tiny amounts of these trace minerals for growth and survival. These amounts can easily be obtained from a typical Western diet. The body has no significant way of getting rid of these minerals once they enter the body, so the addition of iron, copper, or manganese in any multiple-vitamin preparation is not optimal for long-term health. It is well established that vitamin C in combination with iron or copper (and less so with manganese) generates excessive amounts of free radicals that can damage cells and/or reduce the effectiveness of vitamins. In addition, the absorption of these trace minerals in the presence of vitamin C is enhanced markedly in the intestinal tract, which can increase the body's storage of minerals such as iron. Increased storage of free iron (not bound to proteins) in the body can increase the risk of cancer, heart disease, and some neurological diseases such as Parkinson's disease.

Misconception 4: Frozen fruit juices and powdered drinks maintain the stated levels of vitamin C for twenty-four hours when stored in the refrigerator.

Fact: This is not true. Frozen fruit juices and powdered drinks may provide beneficial amounts of vitamin C when drunk immediately after preparation. When they are stored in a cold place and exposed to light and/or air (oxygen), however, the vitamin C in the solution rapidly deteriorates. After twenty-four hours, more than 50 percent of vitamin C activity is lost. Orange juice in cartons may have more vitamin C than the orange juice in plastic containers, but repeated opening and closing diminishes vitamin C levels.

Misconception 5: To maintain good health or prevent cancer, some people believe they should take all their vitamins once a day. Others believe taking micronutrients, such as vitamin C, once in a while (for example, only during a cold) is enough.

Fact: These beliefs may not be true. The frequency with which one should take a multiple-vitamin preparation depends on the rate of degradation of the vitamins in the body. The rate of elimination of micronutrients in the body varies markedly from one vitamin to another; therefore, ingesting micronutrients once a day cannot maintain steady levels of micronutrients in the blood and tissue. Taking micronutrients, including antioxidants, twice a day (morning and evening with meals), however, will achieve a more constant level of these micronutrients in the body. Consuming antioxidants before a meal has the beneficial effect of reducing the formation of cancer-causing agents during the digestion of food (such as nitrosamine with nitrite-rich foods). Taking one or two micronutrients occasionally (for instance, only when one has a cold) has no real health value.

Misconception 6: Avoiding excessive consumption of red meat has no role in preventing cancer.

Fact: Laboratory experiments have shown that this may not be true. For example, excessive consumption of red meat in Western countries has been linked to the development of colon cancer, a finding that is supported by the fact that the incidence of colon cancer among Seventh Day Adventist, a religious group whose members are vegetarians, is extremely low (Fraser 1999). In addition, heme, a component of hemoglobin in the red blood cell, is present in red meat in larger amounts than in white meat and can cause increased proliferation of the cells lining the wall of colon, which can contribute to the risk of cancer. For this reason, excessive consumption of red meat should be avoided in order to maintain good health and reduce the risk of cancer.

Misconception 7: Supplementary micronutrients, including antioxidants, are not useful for cancer prevention.

Fact: This is incorrect and has been propagated by the results of a human clinical study (Albanes et al. 1995) in which a single micronutrient, beta-carotene, was administered orally once a day to individuals at high risk of developing cancer (such as heavy cigarette smokers) for several years. The results showed that the incidence of lung cancer and other cancers increased in the beta-carotene-treated group compared to those who did not receive beta-carotene. The use of one antioxidant alone in this high-risk population has no scientific merit for the following reasons: (a) heavy cigarette smokers have a high oxidative environment in their bodies; and (b) a single antioxidant, such as beta-carotene, will be damaged in such an environment and then will act as a pro-oxidant (free radical) rather than as an antioxidant. Therefore, increased incidence of cancer in the beta-carotene-treated group might actually be expected. Thus, the results obtained from the use of a single antioxidant should not be extrapolated to the effects that can be obtained by the use of multiple-antioxidant preparation in which other antioxidants will prevent conversion of one into a pro-oxidant. On the other hand, there are many laboratory studies and a few human studies that indicate that multiple supplementary micronutrients are essential in lowering the risk of cancer.

Misconception 8: The results of studies on micronutrients and cancer prevention have been published in prestigious peer-reviewed scientific journals; therefore, the recommendations based on such results must be true.

Fact: This may not be correct. For example, if the human studies have been performed on the role of micronutrients in reducing the cancer risk by epidemiologic study (survey-type study), they are important but not sufficient for making a recommendation to the public regarding the importance of micronutrients in cancer prevention. This is because such studies establish only an association between high intake of micronutrients and reduced risk of cancer; they do not establish whether supplementary micronutrients are essential for cancer prevention. Therefore, the results of survey-type studies must be confirmed by laboratory experiments as well as by human studies in which multiple micronutrients, including dietary and endogenous antioxidants, are administered orally daily, for several years, to populations at high risk of developing cancer. Any clinical study in which the efficacy of only one micronutrient on the incidence of cancer, in a high-risk population, has been evaluated should not be used to make recommendations to the public regarding the value of multiple micronutrients in cancer prevention.

Misconception 9: If a single antioxidant is effective in reducing the risk of cancer in animal models, the same result can be expected from using only one antioxidant in humans.

Fact: This belief is incorrect, although many researchers have utilized such an idea in the design of clinical studies in humans. The doses of individual antioxidants needed to reduce the incidence of cancer in animals are generally very high, and the extrapolation to equivalent doses in humans would result in toxic levels of some antioxidants. In addition, the rate of formation and degradation of micronutrients in the bodies of animals may be totally different from that of humans. The fact that the use of a single antioxidant is effective in reducing the risk of cancer in animals but not in humans further supports the idea that the results of animal studies on a single antioxidant and cancer prevention are not applicable to humans.

Misconception 10: A balanced diet is sufficient for optimal protection against cancer.

Fact: Although a balanced diet is necessary in the design of any cancer-prevention plan, it may not be adequate for optimal protection against cancer for the following reasons: (a) the concept of balanced diet is not well defined, and even when it is defined, it is difficult for all individuals to follow in a consistent manner; (b) trying to obtain the optimal levels of antioxidants such as vitamins A, C, and E and beta-carotene through a balanced diet only may not be possible or practical; (c) optimal levels of endogenous antioxidants such as glutathione, alpha-lipoic acid, and coenzyme Q10 cannot be obtained from a balanced diet; and (d) all foods that we consume on a daily basis contain both protective and toxic substances. In order to maximize the intake of protective substances, supplementary micronutrients, including dietary and endogenous antioxidants, should be used together with a healthy diet and changes in lifestyle for maximum protection against cancer.

Misconception 11: Our environment, including food and water, is already polluted, and we have to accept the increased risk of cancer as a part of living in today's world.

Fact: Although it is impossible to remove all cancer-causing substances from our environment, diet, and water, we certainly can lessen their actions with proper supplementary micronutrients and a healthy diet and lifestyle.

Misconception 12: Large amounts of zinc are necessary for optimal health and cancer prevention.

Fact: Small amounts of zinc are essential for our survival. Many important biological reactions in the body require zinc for their activity; however, excess zinc may block the absorption of selenium, an important anticancer agent, and may impair the function of mitochondria. The normal function of mitochondria is essential for generating energy. Impaired mitochondria are associated with some neurological ailments such as Alzheimer's disease and Parkinson's disease.

Misconception 13: Cancer is a disease of old people, so you don't have to worry as much about children following a cancer-preventing diet.

Fact: Although this may be true for some cancers (such as colon cancer and prostate cancer), many cancers can develop at any age. Thus, micronutrient supplementation and changes in diet and lifestyle are also important for children.

Misconception 14: We cannot do anything about reducing the risk of cancer in individuals who have a familial risk of developing certain types of cancer.

Fact: In view of recent laboratory experiments, this idea may not be correct. Insertion of a cancer-causing gene (mutated HOP-TUM-1) in female fruit flies makes them very vulnerable to developing the disease. The incidence of cancer in these flies is markedly enhanced by proton radiation (a form of ionizing radiation associated with cosmic radiation at high altitude, such as on the moon surface); however, supplementation with antioxidants through diet prevents radiation-induced cancer in these flies. Although these results cannot be readily extrapolated to humans, they suggest that the familial (inherited) risk of developing cancer could be reduced through micronutrient supplementation.

Misconception 15: Most supplementary micronutrients, including antioxidants, pass out of the body in the urine and feces, so taking them isn't useful.

Fact: This belief is incorrect. There is no doubt that consumption of high doses of micronutrients can lead to increased levels of them and their degraded products in the urine and feces. But the beneficial actions of these micronutrients are also performed during the digestion of food. The absorption from the intestinal tract of most orally ingested antioxidants, at moderate doses, is about 10 percent; however, the presence of the remaining amounts of antioxidants in the intestinal tract perform very important beneficial functions. For example, increased amounts of vitamins C and vitamin E (alpha-tocopherol) are needed in the stomach to prevent the formation of nitrosamine, a potent cancer-causing agent that is formed from nitrite-containing foods such as bacon, sausage, hot dogs, or cured meat. These antioxidants can reduce the levels of toxins (mutagens that alter genetic activity and increase the risk of cancer) formed during digestion in the intestinal tract. For these reasons, higher-than-normal amounts of antioxidants in the urine and feces should not be considered wasteful, since they produce beneficial effects in the body even without being completely absorbed.

Misconception 16: Supplementary vitamin C causes kidney stones.

Fact: This effect of vitamin C has not been observed in normal individuals even at high doses. The link between vitamin C intake and kidney stones is derived from two observations: (1) people taking high doses of vitamin C sometimes show increased excretion of oxalic acid in the urine; and (2) many people who have kidney stones also have higher-than-normal levels of oxalic acid in the urine. These two observations may reflect independent biological events that are not always associated with the disease. In addition, there are no published reports to support the conclusion that high doses of vitamin C produce kidney stones in healthy individuals. The body normally neutralizes any acidic solution it takes in. If the urine becomes acidic, this suggests that the blood has reduced capacity to neutralize acid. In the presence of an acidic environment, some of the waste products in the kidney may solidify to form kidney stones. Therefore, in certain specific conditions in which one's body has lost the capacity to neutralize acidic solutions, one should not take vitamin C in large amounts.

Misconception 17: Since antioxidants block the capacity of the endogenous antioxidant response after exposure to increased oxidative stress (excessive amounts of free radicals), taking antioxidants may be harmful to your health.

Fact: When the body is exposed to increased oxidative stress, the amounts of antioxidant enzymes become elevated to neutralize the action of free radicals. Pretreatment with antioxidants does not allow the elevation of antioxidant enzymes after exposure to increased oxidative stress. This is often interpreted to mean that antioxidants block the normal response of the body to meet the challenge of increased oxidative stress, and, therefore, could be harmful. This is an incorrect interpretation of the results. A more scientifically rational interpretation would be that antioxidants prevent oxidative stress; therefore, there is no need for the body to respond.

Misconception 18: Beta-carotene acts only as a parent of vitamin A and has no other function of its own.

Fact: Based on recent studies, this statement is incorrect. In addition to acting as a parent of vitamin A (one molecule of beta-carotene produces two molecules of vitamin A), beta-carotene has some biological effects that vitamin A does not. For example, beta-carotene enhances the expression of the connexin gene, which produces gap junction proteins in cancer cells, but vitamin A has no such effect. A gap junction protein is important in holding two normal cells together. Induction of this protein suggests that some cancer cells can become more like normal cells. Vitamin A is necessary for the differentiation of normal cells to various cell types in the body during development, whereas beta-carotene does not have this effect. There are other differences in action between vitamin A and beta-carotene on cancer and normal cells. Since they have different modes of action, the addition of both vitamin A and beta-carotene into multiple-vitamin preparations for cancer prevention is important. Unfortunately, the addition of beta-carotene is discouraged by the establishment at this time for fear that it may increase the risk of cancer.

Misconception 19: All fat-soluble antioxidants consumed at doses higher than RDA (recommended daily allowances) are toxic to humans.

Fact: This is not true for all fat-soluble antioxidants. Only vitamin A when taken at high doses over a long period of time or during pregnancy has been shown to be toxic. Vitamin E at high doses over a long period of time can increase the risk of bleeding in some individuals.

Misconception 20: Natural and synthetic antioxidants have similar effects on cancer cells.

Fact: Various organs in our body selectively absorb the natural form of vitamin E over the synthetic form. Natural beta-carotene can reduce the formation of radiation-induced cancer cells, whereas synthetic beta-carotene cannot.

Misconception 21: Antioxidants have one and only one function in normal and cancer cells: they protect them from free-radical damage.

Fact: In addition to destroying free radicals, antioxidants have some biological effects that are independent of antioxidant activity, such as gene regulation and induction of differentiation in cancer cells (converting them to normal-like cells in some cases). The effect of antioxidants on cancer cells depends on the dose of antioxidant and period of treatment.

Misconception 22: It is not possible for antioxidants to protect against damage produced by different types of harmful agents, such as radiation, toxic chemicals, and pathogenic viruses and bacteria.

Fact: Radiation (such as X-rays and gamma rays) and certain toxic chemicals (such as mustard gas and chlorine gas) cause the most damage to cells by producing excessive amounts of free radicals and acute or chronic inflammation. Among known prescription and nonprescription drugs, antioxidants are the only group of nutrients that can destroy free radicals, decrease acute and chronic inflammation, and stimulate immune function. A good immune system is necessary to prevent and recover from infection with harmful viruses or bacteria. Therefore, antioxidant-induced stimulation of the immune system will reduce the risk of infection by harmful microorganisms.

Misconception 23: Micronutrients alone are sufficient to treat all cancers.

Fact: Because of the complexities of cancer cells, no antioxidants, individually or in combination, are sufficient to treat cancer. However, intravenous infusion of extremely high doses of vitamin C has been shown to be of some value in extending the life span of individuals who have become unresponsive to standard cancer therapy. Using micronutrients in the treatment of cancer (during or after therapy) must be done according to scientific rationale and in consultation with oncologists who have knowledge of micronutrients; otherwise they may be ineffective or even harmful.

Misconception 24: High doses (therapeutic doses) and low doses (preventive doses) of antioxidants have similar effects on normal and cancer cells.

Facts: Therapeutic doses of antioxidants have been shown to inhibit the growth of cancer cells but have no such effect on normal cells. On the other hand, preventive doses of antioxidants generally have no effect on normal or cancer cells.

Misconception 25: Therapeutic doses of antioxidants alone or in combination may actually protect cancer cells during radiation therapy or chemotherapy.

Fact: Laboratory experiments have shown that therapeutic doses of dietary antioxidants such as vitamins A, C, and E and beta-carotene alone or in combination can increase the effect of radiation therapy and chemotherapy on cancer cells, but not on normal cells. On the other hand, administration of endogenous antioxidants such as glutathione-elevating agents (n-acetylcysteine and alpha-lipoic acid) may protect both normal cells and cancer cells. A few clinical studies published on this issue (see chapter 8) suggest that therapeutic doses of dietary antioxidants do not protect cancer cells during radiation therapy or chemotherapy. The value of therapeutic doses of antioxidants remains controversial, and most oncologists do not recommend them.

CONCLUDING REMARKS

At this time, many misconceptions exist about the value of micronutrients, including dietary and endogenous antioxidants, in health care and in cancer prevention and treatment. A few have been discussed in this chapter. Addressing these misconceptions is a challenge for researchers, physicians, and other health care professionals. Improving the health of the general population depends on the success of educating health care professionals and others about these misconceptions. Addressing these misconceptions is equally important in order to promote the correct utilization of micronutrient supplements for optimal health and cancer prevention and treatment. We recommend that you combine a scientifically based multiple-micronutrient preparation containing antioxidants with a balanced diet and changes in lifestyle for optimal health and prevention and treatment of cancer, founded on both the information in this book and consultation with your doctors and health care professionals.

2 The Real Facts about Cancer

Damage to genetic material can increase the risk of cancer. The human genome (genetic material of the human body) contains about fifty thousand genes, but only about five thousand genes are considered active. This genetic material sustains about ten thousand mutations (changes in gene activity) per day as it is exposed to mutagens (agents altering gene activity) and carcinogens (cancer-causing substances) from environmental, dietary, and lifestyle-related factors. One of the consequences of such exposure is the development of cancer. Most cancers occur spontaneously and can develop at any age; however, a few hereditary tumors (tumors that are due to inherited genes) often arise at an early age. Some cancers are related to gender, such as prostate cancer in men and ovarian and cervical cancer in women. Some cancers develop more commonly at certain ages, such as colon cancer in older people and neuroblastoma (a cancer of embryonic nerve cells) in children and Wilms' tumor (a tumor of the kidney) in younger people. Many cancers, however, can appear at any age.

There is also regional variation in the types and incidence of cancer around the world. In Western industrialized nations, such as the United States and the European Union, the predominant types of cancer include breast, colon, lung, and prostate. In the industrialized nations of the East, such as Japan, the incidence of breast cancer is lower, but the incidence of gastric and liver cancer is higher. In other areas, such as India, the Middle East, and China, the incidence of gastric, liver, and cervical cancer is higher. The incidence of lung cancer is high in many regions because of the prevalence of smoking (Prasad 2011).

INCIDENCE OF CANCER IN THE UNITED STATES

In spite of extensive research on cancer prevention during the past several decades, the incidence of cancer appears to be on rise (Table 2.1), having increased from 1.2 million new cases per year to about 1.5 million new cases per year over the course of a decade.

TABLE 2.1. INCIDENCE OF NEW CASES OF CANCER IN THE UNITED STATES PER YEAR (IN MILLIONS)

Year	Men	Women	Total
2009*	0.77	0.71	1.48
2008**	0.75	0.69	1.44
A decade ago			1.2

*Estimated by the American Cancer Society.
**Estimated by the U.S. Mortality Data 2005, National Center for Health Statistics, Center for Disease Control and Prevention, 2008.

The incidence of prostate cancer represents about 25 percent of all cancers, breast cancer about 27 percent, lung cancer 14 to 15 percent, and colon and rectal cancer about 10 percent. During the period of 2003 to 2005, the American Cancer Society estimated that the lifetime probability of developing all types of cancer is 1 in 2 in men and 1 in 3 in women; for prostate cancer, 1 in 6; for breast cancer, 1 in 8; for lung cancer, 1 in 13 in men and 1 in 16 in women; and for colon and rectal cancer, 1 in 18 in men and 1 in 20 in women.

Cancer Mortality

The U.S. mortality rate from cancer has not changed significantly during the past several decades, despite extensive research and development of new treatment methods and drugs (Table 2.2).

TABLE 2.2. CHANGES IN
CANCER MORTALITY SINCE 1950

Year	Death rate per 100,000 cancer patients
1950	194
1991	251
2005	184
2006	181

From K. N. Prasad, *Micronutrients in Health and Disease*, Boca Raton, Fla.: Francis and Taylor Publishing Groups, 2011.

The cancer death rate data from 1991 may be abnormally high (251 deaths per 100,000 patients) compared with those in 2005 and 2006 (181 and 184 deaths per 100,000 patients). Thus, it appears that cancer deaths in 2005 and 2006 were reduced markedly compared to those in 1991, but they were not reduced significantly compared to those in 1950 (194 deaths per 100,000). It is more likely that the cancer death rate that increased between 1950 and 1991 was later prevented through advancement of current treatments. The reasons for the rise in cancer deaths in 1991 are unknown.

In 2003 and 2004 the total deaths from all cancers were 552,888; in 2006 they were 559,888; and in 2009 they were 562,340. These data show that there was a progressively small increase in cancer mortality—of 7,000 deaths in 2006 compared to that in 2003, and an increase of 2,452 deaths in 2009 compared to that in 2006. Deaths from lung cancer were highest in men (30 percent), compared to 26 percent in women. Deaths from other cancers include 9 percent from prostate cancer in men, 15 percent from breast cancer in women, and 9 percent from colon and rectal cancer in both men and women. About 26 percent of all male deaths and 23 percent of all female deaths were due to cancer.

The above data on cancer incidence and mortality suggests that the incidence of new cancer is increasing, while there is no significant change in death rates from cancer since 1950. On the contrary, there appears to have been a slight increase in cancer deaths since 2003. An effective cancer-prevention strategy remains one of the most hopeful approaches to reduce the incidence of cancer in humans. In addition, new treatment approaches are needed to reduce death rates from cancer.

Cost of Cancer

In 2009 the National Institutes of Health estimated that the overall annual direct and indirect cost of cancer in 2008 was $228.1 billion. This cost included $93.2 billion for medical expenses, $18.8 billion for lost productivity due to illness, and $116.1 billion for lost productivity due to premature death.

WHAT ARE CANCER CELLS?

Tumor is the common term used for both malignant and benign growths of cells. The growth of cancer cells in the body depends on several factors, such as nutritional status and vascular supply. Some tumors, such as certain ovarian and breast cancers and prostate cancer, also use sex hormones for their growth.

Cancer cells divide like normal cells, but unlike normal cells, which regularly undergo differentiation (maturation) and death every day, they continue to divide without restriction and can invade and spread to distant organs in the body. The process of spreading to distant organs is called *metastasis*. When normal cells are grown outside the body in laboratory petri dishes, a procedure known as tissue culture or cell culture, they have a limited life span, and all cells eventually die even when they have adequate nutrients and space to grow. In this sense, normal cells can be considered "mortal." On the other hand, cancer cells will continue to grow indefinitely in tissue-culture petri dishes, provided sufficient nutrients and space are available. In this sense, cancer cells are considered "immortal." Cancer cells can arise in any organ that contains dividing cells (e.g., bone marrow, skin, intestine, breast, lung, colon, and prostate) or that has cells that normally do not divide but will divide if properly stimulated (e.g., liver cells, and glial cells in the brain).

CLASSIFICATION OF TUMORS

Tumors can be classified into two major categories: benign tumors and malignant tumors. Benign tumor cells divide abnormally, form a mass, and grow slowly but do not metastasize (spread to distant organs). Examples of benign tumors are polyps in the colon and fibroadenoma in the breast. A benign tumor, if not removed, can become malignant in rare cases after a prolonged period of time. Malignant tumors can metastasize to distant organs. If they arise from mesenchymal tissue (such as connective tissue, bone marrow cells, and bone), they are called sarcomas. A few examples of sarcomas are osteosarcoma (bone cancer), fibrosarcoma, and liposarcoma (cancer of the fat cells). If malignant tumors arise from epithelial cells (cells that cover surfaces or line cavities in the body), they are called carcinomas. Examples of carcinomas include adenocarcinoma of the lung and squamous cell carcinoma of the skin. Other types of malignant tumors include melanoma (cancer of pigment-producing cells called melanocytes), lymphoma, and leukemia (cancer of the white blood cells). Most human tumors are of epithelial-cell origin. Different tumors spread through distinct pathways. Some migrate to various organs through the lymphatic system and others through the blood vessels. The liver and lungs are common sites for metastases.

MAJOR WARNING SIGNS AND SYMPTOMS OF CANCER

The major warning signs and symptoms of cancer vary markedly, depending on the type of cancer. Some of these are briefly described below.

General: Weakness, fatigue, and significant weight loss
Breast cancer: Persistent lump, bloody discharge from the nipple,

ulcer that does not heal, retraction of the nipple, dimpling of the skin

Lung cancer: Persistent cough, coughing up blood, chest pain

Cervical cancer: Spotting of blood after intercourse, painful intercourse, discharge from the vagina

Skin cancer: Increase in size, ulceration, or change in color of a mole; nonhealing and persistent ulcer

Rectal and colon cancer: Alternating diarrhea and constipation, bloody discharge in the stool, and associated weight loss

Bone cancer: Prolonged pain in the bones without any injury, with or without swelling

Testicular cancer: Persistent, firm swelling in the testis, usually without pain

Hodgkin's disease: Firm and painless enlargement of the lymph nodes, fever, excessive sweating, fatigue

Leukemia: Weakness, loss of appetite, bone and joint pain, fever, lymph-node swelling

HOW DO NORMAL CELLS BECOME CANCEROUS?

The processes of converting normal cells to cancer are very complex in humans. In general, it is believed that when dividing normal cells accumulate several genetic defects (mutations or altered genetic activity) over a long period of time, they become cancer cells. Human tumors have a long latent period (three to thirty years), defined as the time interval between exposure to carcinogens and the formation of clinically detectable cancer. This implies that preventive strategy can be implemented in high-risk populations at any time before cancer becomes detectable. Despite extensive research on the formation of cancer cells, the primary genes that initiate the development of human cancer remain elusive in most cases. Some proposed ideas on cancer formation include activation of oncogenes in normal cells, loss of tumor-suppressor genes from normal cells, and infection with cancer-causing viruses.

Some scientists proposed that the process of cancer formation from normal cells can be divided into two phases: the tumor-initiating phase and the tumor-promoting phase (Boutwell 1983). Agents that can initiate the process of cancer formation are called tumor initiators. High doses of tumor initiators are sufficient to cause cancer; low doses of tumor initiators may not cause cancer unless they are helped by *tumor promoters*—agents that cause tumor promotion. Even high doses of tumor promoters alone generally do not give rise to cancer. This theory of cancer formation has been useful in identifying cancer-causing and cancer-protective substances. Some commonly known tumor initiators and tumor promoters are listed below. Most of them are found in the diet, environment, lifestyle, and workplace.

Commonly Known Tumor Initiators
Nitrosamine
Benzo(a)pyrene
7,12-Dimethylbenz(a)anthracene
Asbestos
Contents of tobacco smoke
Polychlorinated biphenyl
Diethylstilbestrol
Polyvinyl chloride
Pesticides (malathion, parathion, kepone, DDT)
Aflatoxin
Dioxin
Most chemotherapeutic agents
Ionizing radiation (X-rays and gamma rays)
Ultraviolet radiation

Commonly Known Tumor Promoters
Certain hormones, such as estrogen
Excess fat, proteins, or carbohydrates
Saccharine
12-O-tetradecanoylphorbol-13-acetate (found in coal tar)
Extract of unburned tobacco

Surface-active agents (sodium lauryl sulfate)
Iodoacetic acid
Phenobarbital

Human beings are seldom exposed to high doses of tumor initiators or tumor promoters, but they are frequently exposed to low doses of these cancer-causing substances. They are also exposed to varying doses of cancer-protective substances. If the relative amounts of cancer-protective substances in the body are higher than those of cancer-causing agents, the risk of cancer development is reduced. Laboratory experiments have shown that the combined influence of two tumor initiators is more effective in producing cancer than the influence of an individual agent acting alone (Prasad, Cole, and Hovland 1998).

Based on microscopic examination of the progression of cancer formation in a given tissue, we have proposed that normal cells go through three distinct stages before they become cancerous (Prasad, Cole, and Hovland 1998). A diagrammatic representation of this model is shown below.

TABLE 2.3. THE THREE STAGES OF CANCER FORMATION FROM NORMAL CELLS IN HUMANS

First Stage
Mutations in normal cells → Surviving mutated cells (proliferate, differentiate, and die in a normal pattern)
Second Stage
Mutation in differentiation gene (proliferate without differentiation, become immortal cells and form tumor mass, such as adenoma in colon)
Third Stage
Mutation in immortal cells cells → Cancer cells

Mutations in genetic material (changes in the DNA) of cells occur constantly in the body. During the first stage of cancer formation, mutations can occur in normal dividing cells from exposure to cancer-causing substances associated with the environment, diet, and lifestyle; from a deficiency in the natural repair system; or from a deficiency in protective substances, such as antioxidants. These mutations can also occur spontaneously. The mutated normal cells may die or survive, depending upon the severity of genetic defects. The surviving mutated normal cells continue to divide, differentiate, and die similar to the patterns observed in unmutated normal cells. These mutated cells continue to accumulate additional mutations at a higher rate but continue for a long period of time to divide, differentiate, and die like unmutated, normal dividing cells.

During the second stage of cancer formation, more mutations occur. When mutations occur in specific genes that are responsible for inducing differentiation, the mutated cells continue to divide without achieving differentiation and subsequent cell death. Such cells become "immortal" and form precancerous or benign growths such as polyps in the colon. These cells continue to proliferate to form a mass.

During the third stage of cancer formation, the "immortal" cells continue to accumulate additional mutations. Most of these mutations play no role in converting immortal cells to cancer cells; however, when mutations occur in specific cellular genes, such as oncogenes (cancer-causing genes) or tumor-suppressor genes, immortal cells become cancerous.

The above model shows that intervention with cancer-preventive agents can be made at any time during the first or second stage of cancer formation in order to reduce the risk of cancer. Cancer-preventing agents could also be useful, if they are administered prior to cells becoming cancerous, because they can reduce the risk of additional mutations in benign tumor cells. The latent periods (time interval between normal mutated cells converting to immortal cells, and between immortal cells to cancer cells) can vary from a few to many years.

As stated previously, most mutations do not have any significant impact on tumor behavior; however, when mutations occur in certain genes, the cancer cells can become very aggressive and cause distant metastasis. Although several studies have tried to establish the relationship between defects in a particular gene and aggressive behavior of tumors, the results have not been consistent.

FAMILIAL CANCER

Most cancers occur spontaneously. They can be induced by cancer-causing substances that are present in the environment, diet, and lifestyle. However, some cancers can occur at an early age because of family history. These include some breast cancers, retinoblastoma, and some colon cancers.

Breast Cancer Genes (BRCA1 and BRCA2)

Breast cancer can occur spontaneously or can be inherited (generally from the mother). Familial breast cancers tend to occur at an earlier age. Two breast-cancer genes, BRCA1 and BRCA2, have been identified (National Cancer Institute 2009). Both are tumor-suppressor genes; in normal cells, these genes help ensure stability of genetic material (DNA) and suppress uncontrolled growth of cells. Mutations in the BRCA1 and BRCA2 genes have been linked with familial breast cancer and ovarian cancer; women who inherit these mutated genes have a greatly increased risk of developing breast and/or ovarian cancer. Although the incidence of breast cancer in men is very low, the mutation of BRCA1 or BRCA2 also increases the risk of the disease in men. Both men and women who have mutated forms of BRCA1 or BRCA2 may be at increased risk of other cancers as well, such as cervical cancer, uterine cancer, pancreatic cancer, colon cancer, and melanoma in women; and pancreatic cancer, testicular cancer, and the early onset of prostate cancer in men (National Cancer Institute 2009).

We should point out that not every woman who has a BRCA1 or BRCA2 mutation will develop breast and/or ovarian cancer. The presence of these mutated genes simply increases the risk of cancer. A woman who has inherited the mutated form of BRCA1 or BRCA2 is about five times more likely to develop breast cancer than a woman who does not have this mutation. In the United States, mutations of BRCA1 and BRCA2 account for 5 to 10 percent of breast cancers and 10 to 15 percent of ovarian cancers among white women. Not all children of people who have mutated forms of BRCA1 or BRCA2 will inherit these mutated genes (National Cancer Institute 2009).

Blood tests are available to check for BRCA1 and BRCA2 mutations. The cost of genetic testing in the United States can vary from several hundred to several thousand dollars.

At present, there are some options available for individuals who have tested positive for the BRCA1 or BRCA2 mutation. They include:

1. **Surveillance:** Screening methods for breast cancer involve mammography and/or MRI (magnetic resonance imaging), and clinical breast examination. For ovarian cancer, screening methods involve transvaginal ultrasound, blood tests for the CA-125 antigen, and clinical examination.

2. **Prophylactic surgery:** Removal of both breasts, and the fallopian tubes and ovaries. Removal of these tissues does not guarantee against developing cancer.

3. **Risk avoidance:** High blood levels of estrogen increase the risk of breast cancer; therefore, the FDA has recommended that hormone replacement therapy (HRT) be used only at the lowest doses for the shortest period of time needed to reduce the discomfort of menopause. It is very important for women to consult their doctors when deciding to take HRT because of its increased risk of cancer.

4. **Lifestyle and diet:** Obesity, lack of physical activity, and excessive consumption of alcohol or dietary fat may increase the risk of breast cancer, and, therefore, they should be avoided.

5. **Preventing agents:** Tamoxifen and raloxifene are FDA-approved drugs that are useful in reducing the risk of breast cancer in high-risk populations (Vogel et. al. 2010; Ntukidem et al. 2008); however, in some individuals, tamoxifen increases cholesterol levels and the risk of stroke, which can be prevented by supplementation with antioxidants such as vitamins E and C

(Babu et al. 2000). In addition, a low-fat and high-fiber diet with plenty of fruits and vegetables can also reduce the risk of breast cancer in high-risk populations. Supplementation with multiple micronutrients containing dietary and endogenous antioxidants may also be important for reducing the risk of cancer.

Retinoblastoma

Retinoblastoma is a tumor of the eye. It occurs in early childhood and accounts for about one case of tumor in every twenty thousand children. The average annual incidence of retinoblastoma in the United States is 5.8 per million under the age of ten years and 11.8 per million under the age of five years. The tumor develops from an immature retina (the part of the eye responsible for detecting light and color). Retinoblastoma can occur spontaneously or can be inherited from a family member who had this tumor. In the familial form of retinoblastoma, multiple tumors are found in both eyes, while in the spontaneously occurring form, only one tumor is present in one eye.

Initially, a gene was identified in the familial form of retinoblastoma. This gene acts as a tumor suppressor and is present in all cells of the body. In retinoblastoma this gene is lost. The loss of or mutation in this gene increases the risk of developing a second cancer. Ninety percent of individuals who have lost or have a mutated form of the retinoblastoma gene will develop this tumor (Aerts et al. 2006).

Retinoblastoma, if not treated, is fatal. The early diagnosis and modern methods of treatments (radiation therapy and chemotherapy) have produced a more than 90-percent cure rate. Unfortunately, about 51 percent of patients with familial retinoblastoma will develop a second cancer within five decades of initial radiation therapy. In addition, the risk of vision loss is high after therapy.

Colon Cancer

Colon cancer can occur spontaneously (most cases) or can be inherited. There are two forms of familial colon cancer: familial adenomatous polyposis and familial non-polyposis colorectal cancer. In case of familial adenomatous polyposis, individuals may have hundreds to thousands of colon polyps at a young age. Both familial forms of polyps increase the risk of colon cancer. Generally, the more family members affected and the earlier the age of diagnosis, the greater the risk of developing colon cancer. If you have a sibling or parent who has been diagnosed with colon cancer, your own risk of developing this cancer is about 1.7 times greater than for individuals who have no family history of colon cancer. On the other hand, if you have two immediate family members with colon cancer, your risk of developing this tumor is 2.7 times greater than for individuals who have no family history of the disease.

MISINTERPRETATION OF LABORATORY DATA ON CANCER-CAUSING SUBSTANCES FOR HUMANS

In laboratory experiments involving cells growing in dishes or using animals, a single tumor initiator, alone or in combination with a tumor promoter, is commonly used for the study of cancer formation. A high dose of these agents is needed to cause cancer. The relevance of this observation to human cancer is often ignored on the grounds that humans are never exposed to such high levels of tumor initiators or tumor promoters. In the real world humans are exposed to many tumor initiators and promoters at very low doses over a long period of time. Laboratory experiments have shown that these potential carcinogens interact with each other synergistically to produce tumors; for this reason the significance of laboratory data on high doses of cancer-causing substances should not be ignored, and every effort must be made to reduce exposure to all carcinogens identified by laboratory experiments.

How to Interpret Human Cancer Studies
To study the relationship of potential carcinogens and cancer in humans, we rely on studies in which we recruit humans who are normally exposed to potential cancer-causing substances or cancer-protective substances from the environment, diet, and lifestyle. The incidence of cancer in this group is compared with those who are not exposed to

the same agent during the period of study. This type of study is called an epidemiologic study (survey type). Epidemiologic experiments are the only tool available to study the association of potential carcinogens with human cancer, because humans cannot be used directly to study the effect of a potential carcinogen on cancer formation. Epidemiologic experiments represent a powerful and useful method for establishing an association between potential carcinogens and the risk of cancer; this type of human study was responsible for establishing the association between tobacco smoking and lung cancer in the 1960s. This association was subsequently confirmed by the laboratory experiments. It is misleading and incorrect, however, to interpret epidemiologic studies to mean that a potential carcinogen identified by these experiments actually causes cancer in humans. Epidemiologic findings must be confirmed by laboratory experiments on human cells or on animal models before such potential carcinogens are designated as human carcinogens.

CONCLUDING REMARKS

Despite extensive research on cancer formation and prevention, the cancer death rate increased between 1950 and 1991; however, in 2006 the death rate was similar to that observed in 1950. This suggested that rise in cancer death rate was prevented by current treatment modalities.

The genetic material in normal cells goes through a series of mutations that take several years to become cancer cells. Several tumor-initiating and tumor-promoting agents have been identified in the environment, lifestyle, and diet. Thus, we can work to limit our exposure to these carcinogens in order to reduce the risk of cancer. Epidemiologic studies are the only way to establish an association between a potential carcinogen and risk of cancer in humans; however, this association must be confirmed by laboratory experiments in which a potential carcinogen actually causes cancer. If epidemiologic studies are not properly performed and interpreted, they can cause confusion among the public about which factors play significant roles in causing or increasing the risk of cancer. These studies are often interpreted as a cause and effect, rather than an association.

3 Free Radicals, Inflammation, the Immune System, and Antioxidants

Before discussing the reduction in cancer incidence or improvement in treatment, we must become familiar with some facts about free radicals, inflammation, and the immune system that play key roles in the initiation and progression of cancer (Cotran, Kumar, and Collins 1999; Pryor 1994; Prasad 2011).

HISTORY, SOURCES, AND PRODUCTION OF FREE RADICALS

In the beginning Earth's atmosphere had no oxygen. Anaerobic microorganisms, which can live without oxygen, thrived. About 2.5 billion years ago, blue-green algae in the ocean acquired the ability to split water (H_2O) into hydrogen (H) and oxygen (O_2). This chemical reaction initiated the gradual release of oxygen into the atmosphere. The increased levels of atmospheric oxygen led to the extinction of many anaerobic microorganisms, for which oxygen was toxic. This important atmospheric chemical event forced organisms to acquire antioxidant systems to protect against oxygen toxicity. Those who succeeded in developing antioxidant systems survived and continue to thrive and participate in the evolutionary processes that ultimately led to the evolution of humans, who utilize oxygen for survival and have complex antioxidant defense system. Free radicals are generated as a by-product of using oxygen. Today the amount of oxygen in dry air is about 21 percent, and in water it is about 34 percent.

As previously stated, free radicals, symbolized by a dot •, are atoms, molecules, or ions with unpaired electrons and can be derived either from oxygen or nitrogen. In 1900 the first organic free radical, triphenylmethyl radical, was identified by Moses Gomberg of the University of Michigan in the United States.

Free radicals are very damaging to all cellular structures, such as DNA (deoxyribonucleic acid), RNA (ribonucleic acid), proteins, fat, and membranes. Our body produces different types of free radicals, most of which are very short-lived. The half-lives of various free radicals vary from 10^{-9} seconds to days. For example, hydroxyl free radicals last for 10^{-9} seconds, superoxide anion for 10^{-5} seconds, lipid peroxyl free radical for 7 seconds, semiquinone free radicals for days, nitric oxide for about 1 second, and hydrogen peroxide for minutes (Prasad 2011). This means most free radicals are quickly destroyed after causing damage.

The sources and methods of production of free radicals are different. Increased oxidative stress from production of excessive amounts of free radicals derived from oxygen and nitrogen plays an important role in human diseases, including cancer. To understand the role of free radicals and antioxidants in the human body, it is important to grasp the relationship between oxidation and reduction processes, which are constantly taking place in the body.

Oxidation and Reduction Processes

Oxidation is a process in which an atom or molecule gains oxygen, loses hydrogen, or loses an electron. For example, carbon gains oxygen during oxidation and becomes carbon dioxide. A superoxide radical loses an electron during the oxidation process and becomes oxygen. Thus an oxidizing agent is an atom or molecule that changes another chemical by adding oxygen to it or by removing an electron or hydrogen from it. Examples of oxidizing agents include free radicals, X-rays, and ozone (Prasad 2011).

Reduction is a process in which an atom or molecule loses oxygen, gains hydrogen, or gains an electron. For example, carbon dioxide loses oxygen and becomes carbon monoxide, carbon gains hydrogen and becomes methane, and oxygen gains an electron and becomes a superoxide anion. Thus a reducing agent is an atom or molecule that changes another chemical by removing oxygen from it or by adding an electron or hydrogen to it. All antioxidants can be considered reducing agents. If the body's environment favors reduction processes, the risk of developing cancer may be decreased (Prasad 2011).

Many other radical species can be formed by biological reactions in the body. For example, phenolic and other aromatic radical species can be formed during metabolism of xenobiotic agents (agents that are foreign to the body, such as the cancer-causing nitrosamine). Furthermore, any antioxidant when oxidized can act as a free radical. Oxidative stress occurs when the generation of reactive oxygen species exceeds the body's antioxidant defense system's ability to neutralize them. Similarly, nitrosylative stress occurs when the generation of reactive nitrogen species exceeds a body's antioxidant defense system's ability to neutralize them.

Processes That Produce Free Radicals

Free radicals are created during the intake of oxygen, during the course of infection, and during oxidative metabolism of certain compounds. Mitochondria are the major sites where free radicals are produced. Mitochondria are elongated membranous structures in the cells that are responsible for producing energy. While generating energy with the help of oxygen, mitochondria produce certain types of free radicals (superoxide anions and hydroxyl radicals) as by-products. During this process about 2 percent of unused oxygen leaks out of mitochondria and makes about 20 billion molecules of superoxide anions and hydrogen peroxide per cell per day (Prasad 2011).

During bacterial or viral infection, phagocytic cells (a kind of white blood cell) engulf invading microorganisms and generate high levels of nitric oxide, superoxide anions, and hydrogen peroxide in order to kill infective organisms. Excessive production of free radicals by phagocytes can also damage normal cells.

In the course of the metabolism of fatty acids and other molecules in the body, free radicals are produced. Certain habits such as tobacco smoking, and some trace minerals such as free iron, copper, and manganese can increase the rate of production of free radicals in the body. Thus the human body is constantly exposed to different types and varying levels of free radicals. Fortunately, we have antioxidant defense systems that protect the body against free-radical damage. This defense system may not be effective if the production of free radicals overtakes the antioxidant system (Prasad 2011).

INFLAMMATION

Inflammation in Latin is *inflammare,* or "setting on fire." The primary features of inflammation at affected sites include redness, swelling, warmth, and varying degrees of pain. These characteristics were first recognized by a Roman physician, Dr. Cornelius, who lived from about 30 BCE to 45 CE.

The cell injury caused by physical agents such as radiation, chemical toxins, mechanical trauma, or infection initiates inflammation, which is generally considered a protective response. However, it can act as a double-edged sword; inflammation is needed to kill invading harmful organisms and for the removal of cellular debris in order to facilitate the recovery process at the site of injury, but inflammation can also damage normal tissues by releasing a number of toxic chemicals. This is an important and highly complex biological response that is tightly regulated and automatically turned off after the completion of the recovery process. During the healing process, the injured tissue is replaced by regeneration of native parenchymal cells, by filling of the injured site with fibroblastic tissue (scarring), or, most commonly, by a combination of both processes. If the damage is not repaired, a chronic inflammatory response is set in motion and is associated with most chronic diseases, including cancer.

Inflammation is divided into two categories: acute and chronic. Acute inflammation occurs following cellular injury or infection with microorganisms. The period of acute inflammation is relatively short lasting, from a few minutes to a few days or longer. Acute inflammation is effective only when the injurious stimuli or tissue are relatively mild. If the tissue damage is extensive or the levels of infective organisms are high, acute inflammatory reactions continue, and consequently the toxic products of these reactions can enhance the rate of progression of damage that may cause organ failure and eventually even death.

Chronic inflammation also occurs following persistent cellular injury and infection. The period of chronic inflammation can last as long as the injury or infection exists. The main features of chronic inflammation are the presence of lymphocytes and macrophages, the proliferation of blood vessels, fibrosis, and tissue necrosis.

Products of Inflammatory Reactions

During inflammation, several highly reactive agents are released. These include cytokines, complement proteins, arachidonic acid (AA) metabolites, and endothelial/leukocyte adhesion molecules, as well as reactive oxygen species (ROS).

Cytokines are proteins produced primarily by activated lymphocytes and macrophages and released during both acute and chronic inflammation. There are different types of cytokines; some play an important role in the repair of cells, while others cause cellular damage. Some examples of cytokines include interleukin-2 (IL-2) and IL-4, which favor growth and tumor-necrosis factor-alpha (TNF-alpha), and IL-6, which participate in cellular damage.

Complement Proteins

During inflammation, twenty complement proteins, including their degradation products, are released into the plasma. They can be toxic to cells (Cotran, Kumar, and Collins 1999).

Eicosanoids

Arachidonic acid (AA) is a twenty-carbon fatty acid that is derived from dietary sources or is formed from the essential fatty acid linoleic acid. During inflammation, AA metabolites, also called eicosanoids, are released. These eicosanoids have diverse biological actions, depending on the cell type. Excessive amounts of these chemicals are very toxic.

THE IMMUNE SYSTEM

The immune system is an important defense against invading foreign pathogenic microorganisms, such as cancer-causing viruses, and is essential for the healing of injured tissues. Foreign antigens or cell injury evokes an immune response that, through the complex processes of acute inflammation, removes the pathogenic organisms and cellular debris. Newly formed cancer cells may act as foreign agents that evoke an immune response, producing natural killer (NK) cells that can remove cancer cells from the body. If there are not enough natural killer cells, newly formed cancer cells can establish themselves in the body and grow.

Antioxidant Defense Systems

The antioxidant defense system in humans can be divided into two groups: endogenous antioxidants that are made in the body, and exogenous antioxidants that are not made in the body but are consumed through diet. Endogenous antioxidants include antioxidant enzymes such as superoxide dismutase (SOD), catalase, and glutathione peroxidase; and compounds such as glutathione, alpha-lipoic acid, coenzyme Q10, and melatonin. Antioxidant enzymes are not effective when taken orally, whereas other compounds are effective taken orally through supplements and/or certain types of food. Standard dietary antioxidants that are commonly used in a multiple-vitamin preparation include vitamins A, C, and E and beta-carotene. Herbal, fruit, and vegetable antioxidants include resveratrol, curcumin, cinnamon extract, and ginseng extract. They are not always added to multiple-vitamin preparations.

The antioxidant enzyme SOD requires manganese, copper, or zinc for its biological activity. Manganese-SOD is present in the mitochondria, whereas copper-SOD and zinc-SOD are present in the cytoplasm and in the nucleus of the cell. They can destroy free radicals and hydrogen peroxide. The antioxidant enzyme catalase needs iron for its biological activity, and it too destroys hydrogen peroxide in cells. The antioxidant enzyme glutathione peroxidase requires selenium for its biological activity and is responsible for removing hydrogen peroxide. Although the trace minerals iron, copper, and manganese are essential for the activities of antioxidant enzymes and other biological activities in the body, a slight increase of free iron, copper, or manganese can amplify the production of free radicals and subsequently increase the risk of cancer. Therefore, it is not a good idea to add these trace minerals to a multiple-vitamin preparation.

HISTORY, SOURCES, AND ACTIONS OF ANTIOXIDANTS

History

Vitamin A

The night blindness that we know now is caused by vitamin A deficiency existed for centuries before the discovery of vitamin A. As early as about 1500 BCE Egyptians knew how to cure this disease. Roman soldiers suffering from night blindness used to go Egypt to receive liver extract for treatment. Now it is well established that liver is the richest source of vitamin A. The treatment of night blindness with liver extract was not used outside Egypt for centuries, perhaps because the medical establishment during that period may not have accepted this treatment. In 1912, Dr. McCollum of the University of Wisconsin discovered vitamin A in butter; it was initially called fat-soluble A. The structure of vitamin A was determined in 1930, and this vitamin was synthesized in the laboratory in 1947.

Carotenoids

In 1919 carotenoid pigments were isolated from yellow plants, and in 1930 researchers found that some of the ingested carotene was converted to vitamin A. This substance was referred to as beta-carotene. There are several types of carotenoids in plants, fruits, and vegetables.

Vitamin C

Scurvy, we know today, is caused by vitamin C deficiency. But the symptoms of this disease were known to Egyptians as early as 1500 BCE. In the fifth century Hippocrates described the symptoms of scurvy, including bleeding gums, hemorrhaging, and death. Native American Indians had a cure for scurvy that included drinking the extract of pine bark and needles (prepared like tea), but it remained limited to their own population for hundreds of years. During the sea voyages of European explorers between the twelfth and sixteenth centuries, the epidemic of scurvy among sailors forced some to land in Canada, where native Indians gave them the extract of pine bark and needles, curing their scurvy.

In 1536, Jacques Cartier, a French explorer, brought this formulation to France, but the medical establishment rejected it as fraud because it came from Native Americans. By 1593, Sir Richard Hawkins began recommending that his sailors consume sour oranges and lemons to reduce the risk of disease. But not until 1770 did the British Navy begin recommending that ships carry sufficient lime juice for all personnel. In 1928, Albert Szent-Györgyi, a Hungarian scientist, isolated hexuronic acid from the adrenal gland. This substance was vitamin C, and in 1932 it was the first vitamin to be made in the laboratory.

Vitamin D

Although the bone disease rickets may have existed in human populations for centuries, it was not until 1645 that Dr. Daniel Whistler described the symptoms, which we now know are due to vitamin D deficiency. In 1922, Sir Edward Mellanby, while working on a cure for rickets, discovered vitamin D. The vitamin later was found to require sunlight for its formation in skin cells, and its chemical structure was determined by German scientist Dr. Adolf Windaus in 1930. Vitamin D_3 was chemically characterized in 1936 and was initially considered a steroid that was effective in the treatment of rickets.

Vitamin E

In 1922, Dr. Herbert Evans from the University of California—Berkeley observed that rats reared exclusively on whole milk grew normally but were not fertile. Fertility was restored when they were fed additional wheat germ. However, it took another fourteen years before the active substance responsible for restoring fertility was isolated. Dr. Evans named it tocopherol, from the Greek word meaning "to bear offspring" and with the ending *ol* to signify its chemical status as an alcohol.

B Vitamins

All B vitamins were discovered during the period of 1912 to 1934. In 1912 the Polish-born biochemist Dr. Casimir Funk isolated the active substances from the husks of unpolished rice that prevented the disease beriberi. He named this substance vitamines because he thought they were "amines" that are derived from ammonia. In 1920 the *e* was dropped when it was discovered that not all vitamins were amines.

Sources of Standard Dietary and Endogenous Antioxidants

Some dietary antioxidants—such as vitamins A, C, and E; carotenoids; and the mineral selenium—will be referred to as standard dietary antioxidants, because they are commonly consumed through supplements. Other types of antioxidants include various kinds of polyphenols found in fruits, vegetables, and herbs, some of which are often added in small quantities to multiple-vitamin preparations. Some standard dietary antioxidants are described below.

Vitamin A

The richest source of vitamin A is liver (6.5 milligrams per 100 grams of liver) from beef, pork, chicken, turkey, and fish. Vitamin A exists as retinyl palmitate or retinyl acetate that is converted into the retinol form in the body, and then into retinoic acid in cells. One international unit (IU) of vitamin A equals to 0.3 microgram of retinol. Vitamin A and its derivative retinoids in natural and synthetic forms are available commercially.

Carotenoids

There are more than six hundred carotenoids in various plants, fruits, and vegetables. Among them, beta-carotene, alpha-carotene, lycopene, lutein, xanthophylls, zeaxanthin, and beta-cryptoxanthin are important. We do not know much about the remaining carotenoids. Beta-carotene, alpha-carotene, lycopene, and lutein have been studied in laboratory experiments and in humans. The richest sources of carotenoids are sweet potato, carrot, spinach, mango, cantaloupe, apricot, kale, broccoli, parsley, cilantro, pumpkin, winter squash, and fresh thyme. One IU of vitamin A equals to 0.6 microgram of beta-carotene. One molecule of beta-carotene produces two molecules of vitamin A. Beta-carotene in natural and synthetic forms is available commercially.

Vitamin C

The richest sources of vitamin C are fruits and vegetables. They include rose hip, red pepper, parsley, guava, kiwifruit, broccoli, lychee, papaya, and strawberry. Each of them contains about 2,000 milligrams of vitamin C per 100 grams of fruit. Other sources of vitamin C include orange, lemon, melon, garlic, cauliflower, grapefruit, raspberry, tangerine, passion fruit, spinach, and lime. These contain about 30 to 50 milligrams per 100 grams of fruit and vegetable. Vitamin C is sold commercially as L-ascorbic acid, calcium ascorbate, sodium ascorbate, or potassium ascorbate.

Vitamin E

The richest sources of vitamin E include wheat germ oil (215 milligrams per 100 of grams), sunflower oil (56 milligrams per 100 grams), olive oil (12 milligrams per 100 grams), almond oil (39 milligrams per 100 grams), hazelnut oil (26 milligrams per 100 grams), walnut oil (20 milligrams per 100 grams), and peanut oil (17 milligrams per 100 grams). Sources for small amounts of vitamin E (0.1 to 2 milligrams per 100 grams) include kiwifruit, fish, leafy vegetables, and whole grains. In the United States fortified breakfast cereals are important sources of vitamin E. At present, most of the natural form of vitamin E is extracted from vegetable oils, primarily soybean. Vitamin E exists in eight different forms: four tocopherols (alpha-, beta-, gamma-, and delta-tocopherol) and four tocotrienols (alpha-, beta-, gamma-, and delta-tocotrienol). Alpha-tocopherol has the most biological activity. Vitamin E can exist in the natural form commonly indicated as "d," whereas the synthetic form is referred to as "dl." The stable, esterified form of vitamin E is available as alpha-tocopheryl acetate, alpha-tocopheryl succinate, and alpha-tocopheryl nicotinate. One IU of vitamin E equals 0.66 milligram of d-alpha-tocopherol, and 1 IU of racemic mixture (dl form) equals 0.45 milligram of d-tocopherol.

Endogenous Antioxidants
Glutathione
Glutathione is formed in the body from three amino acids, L-cysteine, L-glutamic acid, and L-glycine, and is present in all cells; however, the liver contains the highest amount. Glutathione exists in a reduced or oxidized form. In healthy cells more than 90 percent of glutathione is present in the reduced form. The oxidized form of glutathione can be converted to reduced form by the enzyme glutathione reductase. The reduced form of glutathione acts as an antioxidant.

Coenzyme Q10
In 1957, Dr. Frederick Crane isolated coenzyme Q10, and Dr. D. E. Wolf, working under Dr. Karl Folkers, determined the structure in 1958. It is needed for producing energy.

L-carnitine
L-carnitine is synthesized from the amino acids lysine and methionine and was originally found as a growth factor for mealworms. It is pri-

marily synthesized in the liver and kidney. Vitamin C is necessary for the synthesis of L-carnitine. It exists as L-carnitine, a biologically active form, and as D-carnitine, a biologically inactive form.

Polyphenols

Polyphenols are a group of chemical substances found in plants and are also referred to as phytochemicals. They include tannins, lignins, and flavonoids. The largest and the best-studied polyphenols are flavonoids, which include quercetin, epicatechin, and oligomeric proanthocyanidins. The major sources of flavonoids include all citrus fruits, berries, ginkgo biloba, onions, parsley, tea, red wine, and dark chocolate. Resveratrol, which has drawn a great deal of attention in recent years, is found in grape skin and grape seed. More than five thousand naturally occurring flavonoids have been identified from various plants. Flavonoids are poorly absorbed by the intestinal tract in humans. All of them possess varying degrees of antioxidant activity.

Solubility of Antioxidants

The lipid-soluble antioxidants include vitamins A and E, carotenoids, coenzyme Q10, and L-carnitine. The water-soluble antioxidants include vitamin C, glutathione, and alpha-lipoic acid. Fat-soluble vitamins should be taken with meals, to aid absorption.

Commercially Available Antioxidants and Their Distribution in the Body

Carotenoids

Beta-carotene is one of more than six hundred carotenoids found in fruits, vegetables, and plants. It is commercially available in natural or synthetic forms. The natural form of beta-carotene is more effective than the synthetic form. Preparations of natural carotenoids contain primarily beta-carotene; however, other types of carotenoids are also present. Synthetic preparations of beta-carotene contain unknown impurities, the toxicity of which remains uncertain. A portion of ingested beta-carotene is converted to retinol (vitamin A) in the intestinal tract before absorption, and the remainder is distributed in the blood and tissues of the body. About twenty other carotenoids, including the products of a variety of ingested carotenoids, also enter the blood and tissues. One molecule of beta-carotene forms two molecules of vitamin A. In humans, the conversion of beta-carotene to vitamin A does not occur if the body has sufficient amounts of vitamin A. Beta-carotene is primarily stored in the eyes and fatty tissues. Other carotenoids, such as lycopene, accumulate in the prostate more than any other organs, whereas lutein accumulates in the eyes more than any other organs. Synthetic forms of lycopene and lutein are not available commercially. All carotenoids are considered fat-soluble antioxidants and should be taken with meals.

Vitamin A

Vitamin A is commercially sold as retinyl palmitate, retinyl acetate, and retinoic acid and its analogues. Retinyl acetate or retinyl palmitate (a stable form sold commercially) is converted to retinol (a form present in the body) in the intestine before absorption. Retinol is then converted to retinoic acid in the cells. Retinoic acid performs all functions of vitamin A, except maintaining good vision. Retinoic acid and its derivatives are used in laboratory studies because they are readily soluble in fat and thus enter cells easily. Vitamin A in the blood takes the form of retinol and is stored in the liver as retinyl palmitate. Vitamin A exists as a protein-bound molecule. The vitamin A product retinoic acid is stored in all body tissues. Vitamin A is a fat-soluble antioxidant.

Vitamin C

Vitamin C is commercially sold as ascorbic acid, sodium ascorbate (1 gram of this type of vitamin C contains 124 milligrams of sodium), magnesium ascorbate, calcium ascorbate, and time-release capsules containing ascorbic acid and vitamin C-ester. It is present in all cells. Vitamin C enters the blood as ascorbic acid, which can be converted to dehydroascorbic acid, which can be reconverted to ascorbic acid. All mammals except guinea pigs and humans make vitamin C. An adult goat makes about 13 grams of vitamin C every day. Vitamin C can recycle the non-antioxidant form of vitamin E to an antioxidant form. Ascorbic acid supplements at high doses can cause upset stomach in some persons. Sodium ascorbate at high doses may increase the concentration of sodium in the urine, which can lead to chronic irritation in the bladder. Time-release capsules contain additional synthetic chemicals. Vitamin C-ester cannot function as vitamin C until the enzyme esterase removes the ester. For these reasons, we recommend calcium ascorbate, which is buffered and is unlikely to produce stomach upset. All forms of vitamin C are water soluble.

Vitamin E

Vitamin E is a term used for all tocopherols and tocotrienols possessing the biological activity of alpha-tocopherol. Both tocopherol and tocotrienol have alpha (α), beta (β), gamma (γ), and delta (δ) forms. Alpha-tocopherol has the highest antioxidant activity, followed by beta-, gamma-, and delta-tocopherol. In recent years, research on tocotrienols has also revealed some important biological functions. Synthetic vitamin E is referred to as the dl form; the natural form is termed the d form. Vitamin E is commercially sold as d- or dl-tocopherol, alpha-tocopheryl acetate, or alpha-tocopheryl succinate (vitamin E succinate). Alpha-tocopheryl acetate and vitamin E succinate forms of vitamin E are more stable than alpha-tocopherol. Alpha-tocopherol, alpha-tocopheryl acetate, and vitamin E succinate have been widely used in the laboratory and clinical studies.

Scientists have presumed that alpha-tocopheryl acetate and vitamin E succinate are converted to alpha-tocopherol in the intestinal tract before absorption. This assumption may be true as long as the stores of alpha-tocopherol in the body are not completely full; however, if the body stores of alpha-tocopherol are full, a portion of vitamin E succinate can be adequately absorbed. Therefore, it is not necessary that all vitamin E succinate be converted to alpha-tocopherol before absorption. Vitamin E succinate enters the cells more easily than alpha-tocopherol because of its greater solubility. In addition, vitamin E succinate has some unique functions that cannot be produced by alpha-tocopherol. Vitamin E succinate is now considered the most effective form of vitamin E, but it cannot act as an antioxidant until converted to alpha-tocopherol. Laboratory experiments have shown that the solvents of some water-soluble preparations of vitamin E are toxic and should be avoided. Alpha-tocopherol is located primarily in the membranous structures of the cells.

Glutathione and Alpha-lipoic Acid

Glutathione is the most important antioxidant within the cells. Glutathione is sold commercially for oral consumption; however, this is destroyed totally in the intestine. Therefore, oral administration of glutathione does not increase the level of glutathione in the cells and will not produce any beneficial effect in the body. N-acetylcysteine (NAC) increases the level of glutathione in the cells. In the body N-acetyl is removed from NAC by the enzyme esterase, and then cysteine is used to produce glutathione. Alpha-lipoic acid also increases the level of glutathione by a mechanism that is different from NAC and is present in all cells. Therefore, both NAC and alpha-lipoic acid should be added to a multiple-vitamin preparation.

Coenzyme Q10

About 95 percent of energy is generated from the use of coenzyme Q10 by the mitochondria. Therefore, organs that require high energy, such as the heart and liver, have the highest concentrations of coenzyme Q10. Other organelles inside the cells that contain coenzyme Q10 include endoplasmic reticulum, peroxisomes, lysosomes, and Golgi apparatus. Coenzyme Q10 is sold commercially as a time-release capsule or simple coenzyme Q10. It is absorbed in the body as coenzyme Q10 and used by mitochondria to generate energy. It also acts as a weak antioxidant. A comparative study of the efficacy of time-release and regular forms of coenzyme Q10 has not been made. We recommend a regular form. This supplement is fat soluble.

L-carnitine

L-carnitine is made in our bodies, but we can also obtain it from the diet. The highest concentration of L-carnitine is found in red meat (95 milligrams per 3.0 ounces of meat). In contrast, chicken breast has only 3.9 milligrams per 3.5 ounces. It is present in all cells of our body.

NADH (reduced form of nicotinamide adenine dinucleotide)

Nicotinamide adenine dinucleotide (NAD+) and NADH are present in all cells of our body. NAD+ is an oxidizing agent and therefore can act as a pro-oxidant, whereas NADH can act as an antioxidant. NAD+ accepts electrons from other molecules and is reduced to form NADH that can recycle oxidized vitamin E to the reduced form that can act as an antioxidant. NADH is essential for mitochondria to generate energy. NADH is water soluble.

Melatonin

Melatonin is a naturally occurring hormone produced primarily by the pineal gland in the brain. It is also produced by the retina, lens, and gastrointestinal tract. Melatonin is formed from the amino acid tryptophan. Melatonin is also produced by various plants, such as rice. It is readily absorbed from the intestinal tract; however, 50 percent of it is removed from the plasma in 35 to 50 minutes. It has several biological functions, including antioxidant activity, and is necessary for sleep. Melatonin should not be used as a routine supplement.

Polyphenols

These are numerous and present in herbs, fruits, and vegetables. Some examples include resveratrol (in grape skin and seed), curcumin (in spices such as turmeric), ginseng extract, cinnamon extract, and garlic extract. They are generally fat soluble. They are absorbed from the intestinal tract and distributed in all tissues of the body. They are important antioxidants but do not produce any unique biological effects that cannot be produced by standard dietary and endogenous antioxidants. Therefore, addition of any one or more of these antioxidants to a multiple-vitamin preparation is not necessary. They should be consumed regularly through the diet.

How to Store Antioxidants
Carotenoids
Most commercially sold carotenoids in solid form can be stored at room temperature, away from light, for a few years. Beta-carotene in solution, however, degrades within a few days, even in the cold and stored away from light.

Vitamin A
Crystal forms of retinol, retinoic acid, retinyl acetate, and retinal palmitate can be stored at 4°C (39.2°F) for several months. A solution of retinoic acid is stable at 4°C (39.2°F), stored away from light, for several weeks.

Vitamin C
Vitamin C should not be stored in solution form, because it is easily destroyed within a few days. Crystal or tablet forms of vitamin C can be kept at room temperature, away from light, for a few years.

Vitamin E
Alpha-tocopherol is relatively unstable at room temperature in comparison to alpha-tocopheryl acetate or alpha-tocopheryl succinate. Alpha-tocopherol can be stored at 4°C (39.2°F) for several weeks, but alpha-tocopheryl acetate or alpha-tocopheryl succinate can be stored at room temperature for a few years. A solution of alpha-tocopheryl succinate is stable for several months at 4°C (39.2°F), if kept away from light.

Glutathione, N-acetylcysteine, and Alpha-lipoic acid
Solid forms of glutathione, n-acetylcysteine, and alpha-lipoic acid are stable at room temperature, away from light, for a few years. The solutions of these antioxidants are stable at 4°C (39.2°F), away from light, for several months.

Coenzyme Q10 and NADH

These antioxidants in solid forms are stable at room temperature, away from the light, for a few years. The solutions of these antioxidants are stable at 4°C (39.2°F), away from light, for several months.

Polyphenols

These are stable and can be stored in solid form at room temperature, away from light, for a few years.

Melatonin

The powder form of melatonin is stable at 4°C (39.2°F) for a year or more.

Can Antioxidants Be Destroyed During Cooking?

Carotenoids

Most carotenes, especially lutein and lycopene, are not destroyed during cooking. In fact, their bioavailability improves when they are derived from a cooked or extracted preparation—for example, lycopene from tomato sauce.

Vitamin A

Among all vitamins, vitamin A appears to be most sensitive to heat. Routine cooking does not destroy vitamin A in a significant amount, but slow heating for a longer period of time may reduce its potency. Canning and prolonged cold storage also may diminish the activity of vitamin A. The vitamin A content of fortified milk powder substantially declines after two years.

Vitamin E

Food processing, frying, and freezing destroy vitamin E. The vitamin E content of fortified milk powder is unaffected over a two-year period.

Glutathione, N-acetylcysteine, and Alpha-lipoic acid

All three can be partially destroyed during cooking.

Polyphenols

These are not destroyed during cooking.

Coenzyme Q10 and NADH

Both can partially degrade during cooking.

Why We Need Micronutrient Supplements

Adequate amounts of micronutrients, including dietary antioxidants such as vitamins A, C, and E; carotenoids; polyphenols; the mineral selenium; and endogenous antioxidants such as glutathione-elevating agents (n-acetylcysteine and alpha-lipoic acid), coenzyme Q10, and L-carnitine are essential for maintaining health and for cancer prevention. A deficiency in one of these micronutrients can have serious adverse effects on health. The constant use of oxygen in the body generates large amounts of free radicals, which are harmful. Increased amounts of free radicals are also produced during infection and during metabolism of certain substances in the body. Specific trace minerals, such as iron, copper, and manganese, in combination with molecules like vitamin C and uric acid can generate large amounts of free radicals.

The body's own antioxidant defense system may not be able to cope with the large production of free radicals under certain conditions, such as aging and initiation and progression of certain chronic diseases. Therefore, the presence of high amounts of antioxidants in the body is essential to destroying free radicals and increasing immune function. Many harmful chemicals (such as mutagens that alter genetic activity and increase the risk of cancer) are formed during digestion of food. The presence of adequate amounts of antioxidants can reduce the formation of these toxic chemicals. Environmental toxins can induce mutations that can be prevented by antioxidants. High doses of antioxidants regulate gene activity in cancer cells in a way that helps curtail the growth of cancer cells. We must emphasize, however, that many of the actions of antioxidants on cancer cells are not due to their antioxidative actions but rather to their role in regulating gene activity. Thus, maintaining adequate amounts of micronutrients, including antioxidants, in the body is vital to optimal health and cancer prevention.

The highest levels of vitamins A, C, and E are present in the liver, and the lowest levels of these antioxidants are in the brain. The heart and liver have the highest levels of coenzyme Q10. Only about 10 percent of ingested water-soluble or fat-soluble antioxidants are absorbed from the intestinal tract. Some researchers have argued that 90 percent of antioxidants are therefore wasted, but this argument has no scientific merit. During digestion processes many toxic substances, including mutagens and carcinogens, are formed. Meat eaters form these toxic substances more than vegetarians. The consumption of organic food makes no difference in the amounts of toxins formed during digestion of food. A portion of these toxins is absorbed from the gastrointestinal tract and could, over a long period of time, increase the risk of cancer. The presence of increased amounts of antioxidants within the gastrointestinal tract markedly reduces the levels of toxins formed during digestion, and thereby reduces the risk of these toxins on health and the incidence of cancer.

The RDA, which is now referred to as daily recommended intake (DRI) has been established for each micronutrient, and these values are considered sufficient for preventing deficiencies and for allowing normal growth and development. These values may not be sufficient for optimal health and cancer prevention or treatment, however. In addition, most standard antioxidants may not be obtained in adequate amounts from one's diet alone (though polyphenols of various kinds can be adequately obtained from the diet). We believe that moderate supplementation with multiple micronutrients, including dietary and endogenous antioxidants, together with a good diet and changes in lifestyle is needed for optimal health and cancer prevention and treatment. The dosage and type of micronutrients needed depend on a person's age, gender, type of disease, disease risk levels (low or high), and disease stage (early or advanced). These topics are addressed in chapter 7.

How Much of Each Antioxidant Do We Absorb and Retain?

Beta-carotene

Only about 10 percent of ingested beta-carotene is absorbed from the small intestine. Among vegetarians who do not eat eggs or dairy products, most beta-carotene is converted to vitamin A (retinol), whereas among nonvegetarians (who have sufficient stores of vitamin A) such conversion does not take place. The turnover of beta-carotene in the blood is slow.

Vitamin A

Only 10 to 20 percent of ingested vitamin A is absorbed from the small intestine. Normal cells characteristically do not take up more than they need to function. Liver cells are an exception. The ingested retinyl acetate or retinyl palmitate form of vitamin A is converted to retinol in the intestine. Retinol is further converted to retinoic acid in the cells; however, most of the body's vitamin A is stored in the liver as retinyl palmitate. Retinol reaches its maximum level in the blood three to six hours after ingestion of vitamin A and drops to a basal level in about twelve hours.

Vitamin C

Absorption of vitamin C from the intestine varies from 20 to 80 percent, depending on the dose. If one consumes 200 to 500 milligrams of vitamin C, about 50 percent will be absorbed from the intestine. To reduce the formation of cancer-causing substances in the stomach and intestine, certain amounts of unabsorbed vitamin C may be useful. Once absorbed, vitamin C is rapidly distributed throughout the body. As with vitamin A, normal cells do not take up more vitamin C than they need to function. Vitamin C is rapidly degraded in the body.

Vitamin E

Vitamin E can be taken as alpha-tocopherol, alpha-tocopheryl acetate, or alpha-tocopheryl succinate (vitamin E succinate). If the body store of alpha-tocopherol is full, a portion of vitamin E succinate is converted to alpha-tocopherol in the intestine before absorption, but the remaining amount is absorbed without degradation. About 20 percent of ingested vitamin E is absorbed from the intestine and is rapidly distributed in the membranous structures of the cells throughout the body. The maximum levels of vitamin E in the blood appear four to six hours after it is ingested. The turnover of vitamin E in the blood is slow.

Polyphenols

These antioxidants are absorbed from the intestine without significant degradation and are distributed throughout the body. The turnover of phenolic compound in the blood is slow. These antioxidants are consumed through the diet in large quantities (grams); for this reason, supplements of a few milligrams in pills may not be useful.

Glutathione, N-Acetylcysteine, and Alpha-lipoic Acid

Glutathione in solid form is fairly stable at room temperature but is very sensitive to oxidative stress. Increased production of free radicals can diminish glutathione level in the cells. It is a powerful antioxidant inside the cells. Glutathione cannot be taken orally because it is completely degraded in the human intestine. In order to increase the level of glutathione in the body, n-acetylcysteine (NAC), which is degraded only partially in the gut and which raises the level of glutathione in the cell, is recommended.

Alpha-lipoic acid is made in the body. Ingested alpha-lipoic acid is absorbed from the small intestine and rapidly distributed into various tissues in the body. Its product, dihydrolipoic acid, also acts as an antioxidant. Both substances remove metals from the body. Alpha-lipoic acid also increases the level of glutathione in the body.

Coenzyme Q10 and Melatonin

Coenzyme Q10 is made in our bodies, and its level is relatively constant unless cells are damaged. The absorption of coenzyme Q10 from the intestinal tract varies, depending on the preparation. Ingested melatonin is also absorbed from the small intestine, but it is rapidly degraded in the body. This hormone is not recommended as a supplement except for the people who have occasional sleep problems.

Actions of Individual Antioxidants

The actions of antioxidants on cells and tissues are varied and complex. Many believe that antioxidants have only one function, that is, to neutralize free radicals. In view of recent advances in antioxidant research, this belief is incorrect. In addition to neutralizing free radicals, they reduce inflammation; stimulate immune function; participate in several biological processes; and regulate the genetic activity involved in proliferation, growth, differentiation, and immune function. Each antioxidant has some unique function that cannot be produced by others. Therefore, it is essential to add multiple antioxidants to any vitamin preparation that is used for maintaining optimal health or cancer prevention or treatment.

Vitamin A

In addition to destroying free radicals, vitamin A plays an important role in maintaining vision, stimulating immune function, regulating gene activity, embryonic development, reproduction, bone metabolism, inhibiting the growth of precancerous and cancerous cells, and improving skin health.

Carotenoids

Beta-carotene is a parent (precursor) of vitamin A. Carotenes are also known to protect against ultraviolet light–induced damage. Beta-carotene increases the expression of the connexin gene, which codes for a gap junction protein (which holds two normal cells together), whereas vitamin A cannot produce such an effect. In addition, beta-carotene is a more effective destroyer of free radicals in the tissues with high oxygen levels than is vitamin A.

Vitamin D

This vitamin is essential for bone formation and regulates calcium and phosphorus levels in the blood. Vitamin D inhibits parathyroid hormone secretion from the parathyroid glands. It stimulates immune function by promoting phagocytosis. It also exhibits antitumor activity.

Vitamin C

It acts as an antioxidant and participates in several enzyme activities that are needed for proper function of the organs. Vitamin C helps in the formation of collagen, and it also takes part in formation of interferon, a naturally occurring antiviral agent. It regenerates damaged vitamin E to an active form of vitamin E.

Vitamin E

This vitamin acts as an antioxidant and regulates genetic activity and relocates certain proteins from one compartment to another within the same cell. It helps to maintain good skin texture, reduces scarring, and at very high doses acts as an anticoagulant. Vitamin E reduces inflammation and stimulates immune function. Its derivative, vitamin E succinate, exhibits a potent anticancer activity.

Alpha-lipoic Acid

Alpha-lipoic acid is a more potent antioxidant than vitamin C or E. It is soluble in both water and lipid; therefore, it protects cellular membranes as well as water-soluble compounds. It regenerates tissue levels of vitamins C and E and markedly elevates glutathione levels in cells. Alpha-lipoic acid participates in several enzyme activities.

N-acetylcysteine (NAC)

This is not made in the body but can be taken through supplements. N-acetylcysteine increases glutathione levels within cells. This function is important because orally administered glutathione is totally destroyed in the small intestine. At high doses, n-acetylcysteine binds with metals and removes them from the body.

Glutathione

Glutathione is one of the most important antioxidants that protect cellular components. It is needed for detoxification of toxins that are produced as by-products of normal metabolism and certain exogenous toxins. Glutathione also participates in several enzyme activities and reduces inflammation.

Coenzyme Q10

This is a weak antioxidant, but it recycles vitamin E to an active form. Coenzyme Q10 is essential in generating energy within mitochondria.

Polyphenols

Flavonoids are one of the polyphenols that have been studied extensively. They exhibit antioxidant activity and reduce inflammation. They also regulate genetic activity.

Melatonin

Melatonin is important in regulating circadian rhythms through its receptor. It also acts as an antioxidant and reduces inflammation. Unlike other antioxidants, when damaged melatonin cannot be regenerated by other antioxidants. It also stimulates immune function.

Summary of Known Actions of Antioxidants
1. Scavenge free radicals
2. Decrease markers of pro-inflammatory cytokines
3. Alter gene expression profiles
4. Alter protein kinase activity
5. Prevent release and toxicity of excessive amounts of glutamate
6. Participate in several biological processes
7. Induce cell differentiation (converting cancer cells to normal-like cells) and cell death in cancer cells but not in normal cells

8. Induce cell differentiation (maturation) in normal cells during fetal development
9. Increase immune function

A Summary of Antioxidant Functions and Doses

At this time the doses of antioxidants that impart the greatest benefit to human health and maximum reduction of cancer risk are unknown. Nevertheless, 40 percent or more of all Americans take micronutrients on a regular basis, hoping to improve their health. In addition, many people with cancer or other illnesses take these supplements in some form, with or without their doctor's knowledge. Many doctors do not recommend micronutrient supplements for optimal health or cancer prevention and treatment.

When one talks with people who are taking micronutrients on the advice of a salesperson at a vitamin store, health-related magazine, book, or television report, it becomes evident that many are doing so without reference to any scientific rationale. Furthermore, the makers of most preparations of multiple vitamins with minerals have not given sufficient attention to the dose, type, and chemical form of the antioxidants or to the appropriate minerals. For example, most of the commercially sold multiple-antioxidant formulas with minerals include iron, copper, and manganese—or all three. But iron, copper, and manganese when combined with vitamin C generate excessive amounts of free radicals. In addition, in the presence of antioxidants these minerals are absorbed better from the intestinal tract, which increases the body's stores of the minerals. Increased free iron (not bound to proteins) stores in the body have been associated with several chronic diseases, including cancer, heart disease, and neurological disease. Therefore, addition of iron, copper, or manganese to any multiple-vitamin preparation has no scientific merit for ensuring optimal health or preventing cancer. In cases where a person has iron-deficiency anemia, however, a short-term iron supplement with vitamin C is essential to help with iron absorption until the anemia is cured.

Many commercially sold multiple-antioxidant preparations contain heavy metals, such as vanadium and molybdenum. Sufficient amounts of these heavy metals are obtained from a normal diet. The daily consumption of heavy metals over a long period of time can increase the body's stores, because the body has no significant way to eliminate these metals. The accumulation of excessive amounts of heavy metals can be toxic to brain cells. Many commercial preparations of multiple vitamins also include inositol, methionine, and choline in varying doses (30 to 60 milligrams). Such doses of these nutrients serve no useful purpose, because 400 to 1,000 milligrams are obtained daily from the diet. Para-aminobenzoic acid (PABA) is present in some multiple-vitamin preparations. PABA has no biological function in the body, and it blocks the antibacterial effects of sulfonamides. Therefore, patients taking sulfonamides and a multiple-antioxidant containing PABA may experience diminished effectiveness of the drug.

Commercially sold multiple-vitamin preparations often contain n-acetylcysteine (NAC) or alpha-lipoic acid. These agents increase glutathione levels in the cells by different pathways; therefore, in order to increase the level of glutathione maximally, the addition of both in any multiple-vitamin preparation is important. Glutathione is a powerful antioxidant that protects both normal and cancer cells against radiation damage. The consumption of NAC and/or alpha-lipoic acid by cancer patients undergoing radiation therapy or certain types of chemotherapy could be harmful, since glutathione could protect the cancer cells from the desired effects of the therapies.

The addition of both beta-carotene and vitamin A to any multiple-vitamin preparation is essential, because beta-carotene not only acts as a parent (precursor) of vitamin A but also has important biological functions that vitamin A does not. Unfortunately, the beneficial effects of beta-carotene have become controversial because of flawed clinical studies that received wide publicity. Thus, the addition of beta-carotene into multiple-vitamin preparations is discouraged and is not approved by the committee responsible for human studies. Other carotenoids, such as lycopene and lutein, are also important for health, but they can be obtained from a diet rich in tomato (lycopene), spinach (lutein), and paprika (xanthophylls, including lutein) in amounts that are much higher than those in supplements. Therefore, the addition of very small amounts of lycopene and lutein to any multiple-vitamin preparation serves no useful purpose for the maintenance of health or cancer prevention. Higher doses of lutein may be needed for eye health, and higher doses of lycopene for prostate health.

The forms of vitamin E, alpha-tocopherol (present in the body) or alpha-tocopheryl acetate (commonly used in laboratory experiments) and alpha-tocopheryl succinate, should be present in a multiple-antioxidant preparation because vitamin E succinate is the most effective form of vitamin E. Laboratory experiments show that alpha-tocopherol (at doses of 20 to 60 micrograms per milliliter) can increase immune function, but beta, gamma, and delta forms of vitamin E at similar doses can inhibit immune function and are not recommended. Similarly, tocotrienols inhibit cholesterol synthesis; therefore, they cannot be used as supplements for healthy people with normal cholesterol levels. Cholesterol is necessary for maintaining normal function of all cells, particularly brain cells. In addition, coenzyme Q10 formation occurs in the same pathway as cholesterol; therefore, reduction in the level of cholesterol by tocotrienol may also diminish the level of coenzyme Q10, a necessary substance for the generation of energy in the body.

Vitamin C is most suitably taken in the form of calcium ascorbate, because it is not acidic and does not cause upset stomach (as ascorbic acid can). The addition of potassium ascorbate or magnesium ascorbate to any multiple-vitamin preparation is unnecessary.

Adequate amounts of B vitamins (two to three times the RDA value) and appropriate minerals, such as selenium, zinc, and chromium, should be included in a multiple-vitamin preparation. Supplementation with B vitamins and certain minerals except selenium may not be important for cancer prevention, but they are essential for maintaining optimal health.

It is not possible to recommend an appropriate multiple-antioxidant supplement that will be useful to everyone, irrespective of age, gender, general health, and disease status. Therefore, separate multiple-micronutrient preparations specific to these groups should be utilized. This issue is discussed in detail in chapters 7 and 8.

If We Consume a Balanced Diet, Do We Need Supplementary Antioxidants for Optimal Health or Disease Prevention?

The perception of a balanced diet may differ from one individual to another. For example, some people believe that a daily intake of one apple, one carrot, one orange, a few fresh vegetables, a little meat, and some carbohydrate constitutes a balanced diet; other people define it differently, with more or less of these individual foods. Generally, a balanced diet may be low in fat and high in fiber, with plenty of fresh fruits and vegetables. This diet may be sufficient for normal growth and development, but supplementary micronutrients, including dietary and endogenous antioxidants, are important for maintaining optimal health and for disease prevention and treatment. One would have difficulty eating fresh fruits and vegetables daily in the amounts and at the rates that maintain ideal levels of dietary antioxidants in the blood. Also, even if a balanced diet were to be defined and standardized, the same balanced diet cannot be applied to all regions of the world, because dietary and environmental levels of cancer-causing substances vary markedly from one region to another. Furthermore, older individuals have reduced capacity to make endogenous antioxidants. It is necessary to take appropriate supplemental antioxidants in addition to eating a balanced diet. An advantage of taking supplemental antioxidants is that one can do so at the most appropriate time to prevent the formation of cancer-causing agents and limit their carcinogenic effects, such as just before eating food containing nitrites or other cancer-causing substances.

It is now known that many foods (even if grown organically) have naturally occurring toxic as well as protective substances. In fact, 90 percent of toxins come from the diet, and only about 1 percent or less are man-made toxins, such as pesticides that are sprayed over the agriculture products (Ames 1983). A balanced diet alone cannot get rid of naturally occurring toxins and is not sufficient for preventing cancer.

It is vital to ingest certain antioxidants at the right time; otherwise, their effectiveness against cancer is minimized. For example, if taken before or soon after eating nitrite-rich foods (such as bacon, sausage, and hot dogs), vitamin C and vitamin E individually can minimize the formation of nitrosamines in the stomach, but the combination of the two antioxidants is even more effective than the individual vitamins. Taking these vitamins a few hours after such a meal may not be as effective for this particular purpose. In addition, studies have shown that levels of fecal mutagens (a possible source of cancer) in people who regularly eat meat are much higher than in vegetarians (Dion et al. 1982). Vitamins C and E have been found to reduce the levels of mutagens in the feces. For this reason, these vitamins should be taken shortly before or soon after eating a meal. (See chapter 7.)

The intake of absolute amounts of antioxidants may not be an important issue in cancer prevention. Instead, the relative levels of cancer-causing substances present in the diet and the environment and the relative levels of anticancer micronutrients, such as antioxidants and selenium, that are present in the body are crucial in determining a person's potential risk of cancer. Consequently, increased amounts of cancer-causing substances and a high level of exposure to such agents in the environment would require a proportional increase in available anticancer micronutrients, which can be supplied by supplemental micronutrients.

As we mentioned earlier, all types of diets, including those that are defined as balanced or even organic, contain both toxic and protective substances. Some toxic agents, such as pesticides, are synthetic, whereas most are found in nature. The risk of chronic illness, including cancer, may depend on the relative consumption of protective versus toxic substances. If the daily intake of protective substances is higher than that of toxic agents, the risk of cancer is lower. Since we know very little about the relative levels of toxic and protective substances in any diet, we cannot know whether we are consuming higher levels of protective substances compared with toxic ones. To ensure a higher intake of protective agents, it is necessary to take a daily supplement of micronutrients including dietary and endogenous antioxidants.

Risk of Taking Micronutrients

The risk of taking micronutrients depends on doses, forms, and frequency of ingestion and duration of consumption, as well as whether they are taken as a single agent or as part of a multiple-micronutrient preparation. Studies have established that when an individual antioxidant is oxidized (damaged by free radicals), it can act as a pro-oxidant (free radical) rather than as an antioxidant (Prasad 2011). For example, in a study published in a peer-reviewed journal, vitamin C was found to lower levels of the oxidized DNA base guanosine (a form of DNA damage) in human lymphocytes, suggesting that vitamin C protects DNA from oxidative injury (free-radical damage) (Duthie et al. 1996). In the same publication, researchers reported that vitamin C enhances levels of the oxidized DNA base adenine (another form of DNA damage), indicating that the same dose of vitamin C intensifies oxidative injury of DNA. Vitamin C in combination with other antioxidants is unlikely to produce such a dual effect, because other antioxidants will prevent the adverse effect of vitamin C on DNA.

Beta-carotene

The toxicity of beta-carotene has become a controversial issue. A few studies have suggested that taking synthetic beta-carotene, at a daily dose of 25 milligrams alone, can increase the risk of lung cancer among groups of people who are at higher-than-average risk of the disease, such as men who are heavy tobacco smokers (Albanes et al. 1995; Omenn et al. 1996). This was not unexpected, because the bodies of heavy tobacco smokers have a high oxidative environment in which beta-carotene will be oxidized and act as a pro-oxidant rather than as an antioxidant. There are no studies that show that if beta-carotene is present in a multiple-antioxidant preparation it will increase the risk of lung cancer among high-risk populations.

There is no known toxicity of beta-carotene up to doses of 15 milligrams in a multiple-vitamin preparation in normal persons or in high-risk populations. Bronzing of the skin may appear after oral ingestion of beta-carotene at 100 milligrams or more over a few months. Deposits of beta-carotene pigment are found in the eye after long-term consumption of high doses, and excessive pigment deposits can harm the eye; these changes are reversible on discontinuation of the supplement. The other carotenoids, such as lutein and lycopene, are relatively nontoxic at oral doses up to 25 milligrams per day.

Vitamin A

The toxicity of vitamin A has been reviewed in a publication (Prasad et al. 2000). Liver toxicity and skin reactions have been noted after oral ingestion of 50,000 IU per day of vitamin A over a year or more. Some of these skin changes are reversible when the vitamin is discontinued, but liver toxicity can be irreversible. Up to 5,000 IU of vitamin A, taken orally and divided into two doses per day (morning and evening), is unlikely to produce major toxic effects in a normal adult; higher doses of vitamin A have been associated with increased risk of bone fracture in older individuals. Ingestion of vitamin A at doses of 10,000 IU per day can increase the risk of birth defects in pregnant women. Because of these toxicities, the recommended daily allowance (RDA) of vitamin A for adults has been reduced from 5,000 IU to 3,000 IU per day. Retinoic acid and other derivatives of vitamin A should not be consumed orally for general health maintenance because of the toxic effects of these compounds at relatively low doses.

Vitamin C

The toxicity of vitamin C has been reviewed in a publication (Prasad et al. 2000). In most healthy people oral doses of vitamin C of up to 10 grams per day will not produce any detectable toxic effects. Intravenous infusion of vitamin C at doses of 50 grams or more has produced no significant toxic effects on blood profiles of cancer patients. In certain diseases involving the metabolism of iron (hemochromatosis, in which the body has very high levels of iron) or copper (Wilson's disease, in which the body has excessive amounts of copper), or the exposure to high levels of manganese (Parkinson's disease–like syndrome), excessive consumption of vitamin C may be harmful, because vitamin C in combination with iron, copper, or manganese, in the presence of oxygen, generates excessive amounts of free radicals. As mentioned previously, increased urinary excretion of oxalic acid in people taking high doses of vitamin C has been interpreted to mean that this vitamin may increase the risk of kidney stones, since increased excretion of oxalic acid also is found in most patients with kidney stones, but there is no scientific evidence that vitamin C supplementation in a multiple-vitamin preparation at high doses increases the risk of kidney stones or gout in most normal people. We believe that up to 2 grams of vitamin C in a multiple-vitamin preparation, taken orally twice a day, is safe in most normal adults.

Vitamin E

The toxicity of vitamin E has been reviewed in a publication (Prasad et al. 2000). In a large human trial of nine thousand normal adults, the daily oral intake of 3,000 IU of alpha-tocopherol acetate for eleven years did not produce any major side effects, though isolated cases of fatigue, skin reactions, and upset stomach have been reported after ingestion of high doses (more than 1,000 IU daily) for a prolonged period of time. Two thousand IU of vitamin E daily can cause a blood-clotting defect, which is reversible after administration of vitamin K. According to many studies, up to 400 IU of vitamin E in a multiple-vitamin preparation, taken per day, is safe in most normal adults. However, the same dose of vitamin E alone may increase the risk of cancer in a high-risk population such as cancer survivors. This is because the bodies of individuals belonging to high-risk populations have a high oxidative environment in which vitamin E could be oxidized, thus acting as a pro-oxidant rather than as an antioxidant.

Polyphenols

Although polyphenols have no known toxicity at doses used in several laboratory and human studies, the adverse health effects of high doses of these compounds have not been evaluated in humans.

Glutathione, N-acetylcysteine (NAC), and Alpha-lipoic Acid

The toxicity of glutathione has been reviewed in a publication (Prasad et al. 2000). Glutathione is considered fairly nontoxic; however, it cannot be absorbed when ingested orally, because it is totally degraded in the intestinal tract. N-acetylcysteine is commonly used to increase levels of glutathione in the body. Doses of up to 300 to 400 milligrams in a multiple-vitamin preparation are considered safe. High doses of NAC can bind with heavy metals such as lead and mercury and remove them from the body, but if such doses are taken on a regular basis, they can increase the excretion of valuable minerals such as zinc, which can adversely affect health. Like NAC, alpha-lipoic acid is also considered a metal chelator; for this reason, long-term consumption at high doses (300 milligrams or more) may induce deficiency of important metals.

Coenzyme Q10

Oral doses of up to 300 milligrams of coenzyme Q10 have been given to patients with breast cancer (Lockwood et al. 1995) and up to 1,200 milligrams to patients with Parkinson's disease without significant apparent toxicity (Shults et al. 2002). High doses of coenzyme Q10 have been used in the treatment of advanced heart disease without adverse effects (Judy, Folkers, and Hall 1991; Langsjoen, Langsjoen, and Folkers 1990). Doses of up to 200 milligrams in a multiple-vitamin preparation, taken orally per day, are considered safe for most adults.

Selenium and Zinc

The toxicity of selenium has been reviewed in a publication (Prasad et al. 2000). The results of animal studies seem to indicate that selenium is a potent anticancer agent. An antioxidant enzyme, glutathione peroxidase, requires selenium in order to exert its antioxidant action. Selenium in combination with vitamin E is more effective than either micronutrient taken alone. Analysis of dietary intake of selenium and cancer incidence has shown that a higher intake may reduce the risk of cancer, including prostate. In a recent clinical study, supplementation with selenium alone failed to reduce the risk of prostate cancer in high-risk populations; this may be because selenium was used as a single agent. Certain metals, such as lead, cadmium, arsenic, mercury, and silver block the action of selenium.

Commercial preparations of selenium include inorganic selenium (sodium selenite) and various forms of organic selenium. Some studies have reported that sodium selenite is not absorbed adequately, whereas organic selenium, including yeast-selenium and seleno-L-methionine, is absorbed very well (Prasad 2011). For this reason, seleno-L-methionine is most commonly used in a multiple-vitamin preparation. The optimal doses of selenium for health benefits are unknown. In the United States the average dietary intake of selenium is about 125 to 150 micrograms per day, while the RDA value of selenium for adults is 55 to 70 micrograms per day. About 200 micrograms of selenium a day (through diet and supplement) have been reported to be helpful in reducing the risk of cancer in some studies, but other studies have shown no such effect. If an average person consumes 125 to 150 micrograms of selenium each day, a supplement of 100 micrograms of selenium in a multiple-vitamin preparation is unlikely to cause major side effects. High doses of selenium (400 micrograms or more), if ingested every day for a long period of time, may induce dry skin and cataract formation in some individuals.

High doses of zinc are commonly believed to be important for maintaining good health, but this may not be true with respect to cancer prevention. Several laboratory experiments have shown that high doses of zinc block the action of selenium. Furthermore, high doses of zinc can damage mitochondrial function and increase the risk of neurological diseases such as Alzheimer's disease (Prasad 2011). Therefore, doses higher than 15 to 25 milligrams of zinc in a multiple-vitamin preparation should be avoided

Consumption of Vitamins, Cost, and Their Reported Adverse Health Events

In 2009 a National Health Interview Survey estimated that more than 50 percent of adults in the United States consume some form of dietary supplements. In 2007 the sales of dietary supplements reached $23.7 billion. Despite the reporting of the negative results obtained from the flawed clinical studies in which a single antioxidant was used in population at high risk of developing cancer, the number of consumers has not declined.

The number of dietary supplements in the marketplace has risen from about four thousand in 1995 to about seventy-five thousand in the year 2008. In addition, food products such as fortified cereals and energy drinks containing dietary supplements are available to consumers in an unprecedented number.

Since the mandatory reporting of adverse health events went into effect in 2007, the Government Accountability Office (GOA) has found a threefold increase in the number of all adverse health events compared with the previous year. The U.S. Federal Drug Administration (FDA) estimates that the total number of adverse health events related to the consumption of dietary supplements—the majority of them herbs such as ephedra—is more than fifty thousand per year. Dietary supplements also include antioxidants such as vitamins A, C, and E, and carotenoids, glutathione, R-alpha-lipoic acid, coenzyme Q10, and L-carnitine, for which there have been no reported adverse health events for decades. However, adverse health effects were perceived by most consumers to include the above antioxidants. We feel strongly that the reporting of any adverse effects of certain herbs should be specific to those herbs, rather than including them under the broad category of dietary supplements. Similarly, the reporting of adverse effects from the use of a single antioxidant, such as beta-carotene, in populations with a high risk of developing cancer, such as heavy tobacco smokers, should include the information that taking beta-carotene alone may increase the risk of cancer among this population. Erroneous or incomplete reporting of scientific observations creates uncertainties and anxieties in the minds of consumers and health care professionals. In our opinion, supplementary multiple micronutrients, together with changes in the diet and lifestyle, may have a very significant impact in the maintainence of good health and prevention and improved treatment of chronic diseases.

CONCLUDING REMARKS

Free radicals are highly damaging chemicals that are produced in the human body. They are generated through the use of oxygen, in the course of bacterial or viral infection, and in the context of the normal metabolisms of certain compounds in the body. There are several types of free radicals in the body; some are derived from oxygen, whereas others are derived from nitrogen. *Oxidative stress* refers to a condition in which high levels of free radicals are produced, causing damage to the cells. Increased oxidative stress is one of the most important risk factors for cancer.

Cell injury caused by physical agents such as radiation, free radicals, chemical toxins, mechanical trauma, or infection initiates an important biological event called inflammation. While this is generally considered a protective response, it can act as double-edged sword. Inflammation is needed to kill invading harmful organisms and for the removal of cellular debris in order to facilitate the recovery process, but inflammation can also damage normal tissues by releasing a number of toxic chemicals. Acute inflammation may not be involved in the formation of cancer, but acute inflammation that occurs during radiation therapy or chemotherapy can damage both normal and cancer cells.

The immune system is an important defense against invading foreign pathogenic microorganisms such as cancer-causing viruses and is essential for the healing of injured tissues. Foreign antigens and cell injury evoke an immune response that through a complex process, including acute inflammation, removes the pathogenic microbes and cellular debris. Newly formed cancer cells may act as foreign agents that evoke an immune response, producing natural killer (NK) cells that can remove cancer cells from the body. If there are not enough NK cells, newly formed cancer cells can establish themselves in the body and grow.

Antioxidants in our body defend against damage produced by free radicals. Some antioxidants are made in the body, whereas others are consumed through a diet containing fruits and vegetables. Both dietary and endogenous antioxidants are essential for optimal health and cancer prevention. The biological half-lives of most micronutrients are highly variable; therefore, they should be taken twice a day to maintain steady levels of these micronutrients in the body. Most micronutrients are very sensitive to light and should be stored in the dark. In a solid form such as a tablet, most (except vitamin A) are stable at room temperature.

Most antioxidants at certain doses are considered safe; however, some, such as vitamin A, beta-carotene, and vitamin E, at high doses can be harmful after long-term daily consumption. The window of safety for selenium and vitamin A is very narrow. Selenium at high doses, for example, can cause cataracts. We believe that daily supplementation with a multiple-micronutrient preparation containing dietary and endogenous antioxidants, B vitamins, vitamin D, and selenium (but not iron, copper, or manganese) should be useful for maintaining optimal health and for cancer prevention.

Although most adverse health events occur primarily from the consumption of certain herbs, the term *dietary supplements* includes both these herbs and antioxidants, which has created misunderstanding among the general public about the safety of antioxidants. However, vitamins A, C, and E and carotenoids, glutathione, R-alpha-lipoic aid, coenzyme Q10, and L-carnitine have had few reported adverse health events for decades, and these adverse health events only occur when these supplements are taken at very high doses.

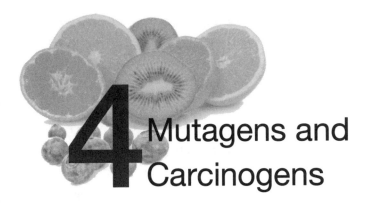

4 Mutagens and Carcinogens

Mutagens are substances that can induce changes in genetic material (DNA) in cells. Although all cancers are preceded by mutations, not all mutations lead to cancer. Carcinogens are substances that actually cause cancer. In order to develop a rational strategy for cancer prevention in humans, it is essential to identify sources of cancer-causing substances (carcinogens and mutagens) in the environment, lifestyle, and diet. Exposure to carcinogens also occurs in the workplace and during diagnosis and treatment of cancer. Studies have estimated that the U.S. diet contributes to about 40 percent of human cancer, tobacco smoking to about 30 percent, the environment to about 29 percent, and familial gene defects to about 1 percent. From these data, it appears that many cancers could be considered preventable (Prasad, Cole, and Hovland 1998).

ENVIRONMENT-RELATED MUTAGENS AND CARCINOGENS

There are numerous carcinogens and mutagens in the atmosphere and work-related environments. These include ozone, ionizing radiation, ultraviolet (UV) radiation from the sun, burning wood and buildings that release high levels of polycyclic hydrocarbons—such as benzo(a)pyrene—asbestos, benzene, and vinyl chloride.

Ionizing Radiation: X-rays and Gamma Rays

X-rays and gamma rays are referred to as ionizing radiation. One environmental source of cancer-causing substances is cosmic radiation (primarily gamma rays), the levels of which increase at higher altitudes. For example, the background level of cosmic radiation in Denver, Colorado, which is located at an elevation of 5,000 feet (approximately 1 mile), is two times higher than that found in New York City, which is at sea level. The environment near uranium mines contains radon gas, a by-product of radioactive uranium. Nuclear testing in the past also has contributed to elevated levels of radiation in the atmosphere, but it is minimal compared with cosmic radiation.

Ionizing Radiation: Neutron and Proton Radiation

Neutron and proton radiation are also called ionizing radiation and are not present in Earth's atmosphere; they are generated by a specialized radiation machine called a linear accelerator. However, at the surface of the moon, proton radiation is high, especially during sun flare-ups. Thus, our astronauts may receive high doses of proton radiation if a solar flare-up occurs during exploration of the lunar surface. Our current technology of predicting the timing of solar flare-ups warns of this event only thirty minutes before it actually happens. Neutron radiation causes damage to tissue via proton radiation. Proton radiation is five- to tenfold more effective at inducing cancer than X-rays or gamma rays (Prasad, Santamaria, and Williams 1995).

Ultraviolet (UV) Radiation and Ozone

UV radiation or light is a part of radiation present in sunlight (also called non-ionizing radiation). Exposure to UV radiation is greater for people who reside at higher altitudes and in areas with a lot of sun throughout the year. Skin cancer, such as the deadly form melanoma, can result from excessive and frequent exposure to sunlight. Melanoma is more likely to develop in people with light skin than those with dark skin; however, the progression of melanoma in dark-skinned people is much more rapid than in light-skinned people. The time interval between exposure to UV light and the formation of a detectable tumor is generally very long, often more than ten years. The use of sunscreen before prolonged sun exposure may lessen the damaging effects of UV radiation on the skin.

Some laboratory studies have reported that the combination of UV radiation and X-rays is about twelve times more likely to generate cancer cells than either type of radiation alone (DiPaolo and Donovan 1976). In addition, tumor promoters present in the diet and environment also may increase the risk of UV-radiation-induced cancer formation and may be partly responsible for a fivefold increase in melanoma incidence in the "sun belt" states Texas, Arizona, Florida, and California. We should note that chemical carcinogens that magnify the risk of X-ray-induced cancer fail to amplify the risk of UV-radiation-induced cancer. Thus, excessive and frequent exposure to sunlight without adequate protection (such as sunscreen and protective clothing) should be avoided in order to reduce the risk of melanoma.

High levels of ozone are found in polluted atmospheres, especially in industrial areas of the United States. The levels of pollution may vary from one day to another in the same area. Breathing ozone can generate excessive amounts of free radicals, which can in turn increase the risk of cancer. Some laboratory experiments have shown that ozone in combination with X-rays increases the risk of cancer about threefold (Borek et al. 1986).

Chemical Carcinogens

There are many chemical carcinogens in our air and water. The air may contain ozone gas, fibers such as asbestos (which was used in insulation decades ago), and chemical particles. The burning of woods in fireplaces, during cooking, or during a forest fire contributes to elevated levels of hydrocarbons such as benzo(a)pyrene, a powerful human carcinogen. The following chemicals can increase the risk of cancer in humans.

> **Dioxin:** a by-product of herbicide and pesticide production and one of the most toxic substances to humans; exposure to only 1 part per billion is hazardous to human health

Polyvinyl chloride: found in packing materials

Pesticides: found as residues on the surface of fruits and vegetables; trace amounts can persist even after washing

Polychlorinated biphenyls (PCB): present in packaging materials and in fish obtained from contaminated rivers

Diethylstilbestrol: a synthetic estrogen often fed to cattle to make them fat

Polycyclic aromatic hydrocarbons, such as benzo(a)pyrene: present in air pollution

Asbestos: found in certain building materials, such as roofing and water-pipe insulation

Aflatoxin: a mold (fungus) found on peanuts and peanut butter if they are not well preserved

Cancer-Causing Viruses

Humans can be exposed to certain viruses that increase the risk of some cancers. They include human T-cell leukemia viruses, SV40 (simian or cat virus type 40), Epstein-Barr, human papillomavirus (HPV), hepatitis B and C, and human immunodeficiency virus (HIV). For example, infection with hepatitis C may increase the risk of liver cancer, HPV can raise the risk of cervical cancer, Epstein-Barr can magnify the risk of certain types of lymphoma (cancer of white blood cells), and HIV can increase the risk of Kaposi's sarcoma (a type of tumor of vascular origin). Laboratory studies suggest that these cancer-causing viruses "immortalize" normal cells and thus initiate a primary event in the formation of cancer (Prasad et al. 1994; La Rosa et al. 1997). The immortalized cells, after some time, sustain specific changes in certain genes, such as cellular genes, oncogenes (cancer-causing genes), or antioncogenes, and then become cancer cells.

Human Papillomavirus (HPV)

Human papillomaviruses are a group of more than a hundred related viruses and are called papillomaviruses because certain types can cause warts, or papillomas, which are benign tumors. About thirty types of these viruses can be sexually transmitted. The types of HPV that cause common warts on the hands and feet are different from those that cause growths in the throat or genital area. Certain types of HPV are associated with a type of cancer and therefore are called carcinogenic, or cancer-causing, HPVs (Chocolatewala and Chaturvedi 2009; Szostek et al. 2009). About six million new cases of genital HPV infection occur annually in the United States. Most HPV infections occur without any symptoms and may go away without treatment over the course of a few years. This may be due to the fact that the immune system will often suppress or eliminate HPV. However, HPV infection may persist for many years in those whose bodies failed to eliminate HPV.

HPV infection is the major cause of cervical cancer (DiPaolo et al. 1993; Franceschi et al. 1996). In 2009 more than eleven thousand women in the United States were diagnosed with cervical cancer and about four thousand died from it. Black and Hispanic women have higher rates of cervical cancer than white and non-Hispanic women. HPV also increases the risk of other cancers, such as vulvar cancer (2,300 new cases per year; rates were higher in white women than in blacks and Asians/Pacific Islanders), vaginal cancer (600 new cases per year; rates were higher in black women than in whites, while Asians/Pacific Islanders had the lowest rates), penile cancer (800 new cases per year; rates were higher in Hispanic men than in non-Hispanic men), and cancer of the head and neck (7,400 per year).

The U.S. Food and Drug Administration (FDA) has approved Gardasil and Cervarix vaccines, which are effective in preventing persistent infections with HPV types 16 and 18. These two types of HPV may be responsible for 70 percent of cervical cancer. Gardasil may also prevent infections with HPV types 6 and 11, which are responsible for 90 percent of genital warts. These vaccines do not treat HPV infections, but they are highly effective in reducing the rate of HPV infection and are considered safe. Widespread vaccination has the potential for reducing the risk of cervical cancer deaths around the world by as much as two-thirds. The greatest benefit of occurs when women are vaccinated before they become sexually active. It is very important for both vaccinated and unvaccinated women to continue to undergo cervical cancer screening tests, such as Pap smears.

Bacterial and Parasitic Infection

Human studies have shown that certain bacteria, such as *Helicobacter pylori,* increase the risk of gastric cancer, the most prevalent type of cancer in some developing countries. In addition, parasites such as *Opisthorchis viverrini* and *Schistosoma haematobium* are considered risk factors for cholangiocarcinoma (cancer of the bile duct of the liver) and bladder cancer, respectively. The eradication of these infectious organisms can lower the risk of these cancers. Chronic irritation, chronic inflammation, and induction of increased rates of division of normal cells may play a role in the formation of some cancers following exposure to infectious agents. In addition, the production of excessive amounts of free radicals and the release of greater amounts of cytokines (chemicals such as tumor necrosis factor-alpha, interleukin-6, and prostaglandins, which can harm cells) during chronic infection may increase the risk of cancer.

EXAMPLES OF LIFESTYLE-RELATED CANCER-CAUSING SUBSTANCES

Alcohol

About two-thirds of American adults consume alcohol, and about 17 percent of them are considered heavy drinkers. Overall, 50 percent of adults eighteen years of age or older are regular drinkers. About 60 percent of men and 42 percent of women are regular drinkers. About 56 percent of non-Hispanic adults are regular drinkers, compared with 42 percent of Hispanic adults and 37 percent of African Americans.

In the United States more than five thousand children under the age of sixteen have had their first full drink of alcohol. The average age at which young people begin to drink is approximately thirteen years. The number of children drinking alcohol is more than those that smoke tobacco or marijuana. The average yearly consumption of alcohol in the United States appears to have declined from 2.76 gallons in 1980 to 2.18 gallons in 2000. The pattern of drinking has shifted from drinking beer to wine, although the drinking pattern of hard liquor has remained the same.

Although alcohol has failed to produce tumors in laboratory animals, the consumption of alcohol has been linked with the increased risk of several human cancers in epidemiologic studies (Genkinger et al. 2009; Homann et al. 2009; Crous-Bou et al. 2009; McCullough and Farah 2008). Alcohol-consumption-related cancers include cancer of the oral cavity, head and neck, liver, larynx, esophagus, colon, rectum, and breast. Excessive consumption of alcohol enhances the cancer-causing effects of tobacco smoking. The combined effects of alcohol and tobacco smoking on cancer risk are about two and a half times greater than the effects associated with alcohol or tobacco smoking alone.

In the Million Women Study at the University of Oxford in the United Kingdom, the relationship between alcohol and cancer was examined in 1.3 million women. The average age of women in this study group was fifty-five years; 75 percent of these women were identified as drinkers, and the period of study lasted for more than seven years. The average alcohol consumption was about one drink per day. The results showed that the risk of cancers of the oral cavity, pharynx, esophagus, larynx, rectum, liver, and breast was elevated in those who drank alcohol. The risk of these cancers increased with the number of drinks, regardless of the type of alcohol. Based on these results, scientists estimated that in the United Kingdom alcohol is responsible annually for about 11 percent of all breast cancers; 22 percent of liver cancers; 9 percent of rectal cancers; and 25 percent of cancers of oral cavity, pharynx, esophagus, and larynx. This study also found that alcohol consumption reduced the risk of some cancers, including thyroid, non-Hodgkin's lymphoma, and renal cell carcinoma (kidney tumor). The reasons for this dual effect of alcohol consumption on cancer incidence are unknown. Although the mechanisms of alcohol-induced cancer are not well understood, some researchers have made the following suggestions.

1. Cancer-causing substances are present in the diet, and they are also formed in the intestine during digestion. Alcohol enhances their solubility and hence the degree to which the body can absorb them. This, in turn, can heighten the risk of cancer.
2. Alcohol may suppress the body's immune system.
3. Alcohol may cause nutritional deficiency, including of antioxidants, thereby raising the risk of cancer.
4. Acetaldehyde, a product of alcohol metabolism in the body, impairs the ability of cells to repair damage to their genetic material (DNA) that may increase the risk of cancer. Alcohol may also activate oncogenes (cancer-causing genes).
5. Alcohol itself is not considered a cancer-causing agent; however, it may act as cocarcinogen and thereby increase the risk of cancer. For example, alcohol consumption combined with tobacco smoking can increase the risk of mouth, tracheal, and esophageal cancer by about thirty-five-fold. Some agents, such as nitrosamine, a cancer-causing substance, do not cause cancer until they are converted into an active form in the liver. Alcohol may facilitate the conversion.

Although higher levels of alcohol consumption are associated with increased risk of some forms of cancer, moderate alcohol consumption (two drinks per day for men and one drink per day for women) may decrease the risk of heart disease and stroke. The benefits of moderate alcohol consumption in heart disease and stroke outweigh the risk of cancer. Therefore, we would suggest that the diet and lifestyle modifications along with micronutrient supplementation recommended in this book for cancer prevention may also reduce alcohol-induced cancer risk, and at the same time may further enhance the beneficial effects of moderate alcohol consumption in protecting against heart disease. All individuals should, of course, avoid excessive use of alcohol and should consult their doctors and health professionals before adopting our recommendations.

Coffee and Caffeine

Epidemiologic studies on the association between coffee or caffeine consumption and the risk of cancer have produced inconsistent results (Ganmaa et al. 2008; Ishitani et al. 2008; Tavani et al. 2001; Song et al. 2008; Lueth et al. 2008; Tworoger et al. 2008; Kurahashi et al. 2008; Larsson and Wolk 2007; Tang et al. 2009). For example, some studies showed no association between coffee or caffeine consumption and the risk of renal carcinoma (kidney cancer). There was no significant association between caffeinated and decaffeinated coffee and tea consumption and the risk of breast cancer. Interestingly, consumption of caffeine-containing beverages was associated with reduced risk of breast cancer in postmenopausal women. In another study no association between caffeine consumption and the risk of breast cancer was found; however, in women carrying a mutated breast cancer gene 1 (BRCA1), which is a risk factor for breast cancer, coffee consumption reduced the risk of breast cancer. Overall there was no association between coffee consumption and the risk of ovarian cancer; however, heavy consumption (five cups or more per day) was associated with increased risk of ovarian cancer in postmenopausal women. On the other hand, another study reported that caffeine consumption increased the risk of ovarian cancer in women on hormone supplements.

Although coffee and caffeine consumption were associated with increased risk of bladder cancer, they were associated with reduced risk of liver cancer. A review of previously published data on coffee consumption and lung cancer revealed that increased consumption of coffee was associated with enhanced risk of lung cancer. Excessive consumption of coffee was associated with increased risk of bladder, pancreatic, and stomach cancer. From these studies it is difficult to draw any specific conclusion about the impact of coffee, decaffeinated coffee, or caffeine consumption on the risk of cancer.

In the laboratory, excessive amounts of caffeine can reduce the ability of cells to repair genetic damage produced spontaneously or by agents such as radiation and chemicals (Puck et al. 1993). Normal human lymphocytes growing in Petri dishes and exposed to low doses of gamma rays (20 mSv) did not shown any detectable levels of mutations. When these lymphocytes were treated with high concentrations of caffeine immediately after irradiation, however, mutations were evident. This study clearly shows that excessive amounts of caffeine can interfere with the repair of radiation-induced genetic damage. Therefore, too much caffeine may enhance the effect of cancer-causing substances and, in this way, act as a tumor promoter.

It is not possible to resolve the controversy regarding the effects of caffeine or coffee on the risk of cancer. In our view, one or two cups of coffee or the equivalent amount of caffeine-containing beverages may have no effect on the incidence of any type of cancer; however, excessive consumption of coffee or caffeine should be avoided in a cancer-prevention strategy. In addition, we suggest that the diet and lifestyle modifications and micronutrient supplementation recommended in this book for cancer prevention may reduce any possible increased risk of cancer from caffeine consumption.

Smoking Tobacco

The U.S. Centers for Disease Control and Prevention (CDC) have estimated that in 2006, 20.8 percent (45.3 million) of adults were cigarette smokers. Of these, about 80.1 percent (36.3 million) smoked every day. Numerous epidemiologic and laboratory studies have confirmed that cigarette smoke is a major human carcinogen (Walser et al. 2008; Ahern et al. 2009; Duan et al. 2009; Johnson, Hu, and Mao 2000; Johnson 2005; Kropp and Chang-Claude 2002; Theis et al. 2008; Hemelt et al. 2009). Smoking tobacco products increases the risk of not only lung cancer but other cancers as well and contributes to about 30 percent of all human cancers. Female smokers have eighty-two times the risk of lung cancer compared with nonsmoking women, whereas male smokers showed only twenty-three times the risk compared with nonsmoking men. The reasons for this marked difference in sensitivity to tobacco smoke are unknown. Chewing tobacco magnifies the risk of oral cancer. Tobacco smoking also can cause emphysema, a serious non-cancerous disease with severe effects on the functioning of the lungs. In addition, smoking increases the risk of heart disease. Although the incidence of smoking is declining among some adult populations, it is growing among teenagers.

What goes on in your body when you smoke? Smoking tobacco releases cancer-causing agents into the body, enhances oxidative damage, and decreases the levels of antioxidants. Cigarette smoke contains a high level of nitrosamine, a potent cancer-causing agent, and nitro-sating gases, which help to form additional nitrosamines in the lungs. Nitrosamines are dissolved easily in water and thus can be absorbed through the mouth as well as the lungs and deposited in other organs. As a result, smoking also heightens the risk of cancer of the larynx, mouth, and esophagus and acts as a contributing factor in cancer of the urinary bladder, cervix, kidney, and pancreas.

Smoking induces several types of oxidative damage that can also increase the risk of cancer. These types include membrane damage (peroxidation), DNA damage, reduced levels of plasma uric acid (an important antioxidant molecule), enhanced adhesion of leukocytes (white blood cells) to the walls of blood vessels, increased aggregation of platelets (blood cells responsible for clotting), dysfunction of endothelial cells (which line the inner wall of blood vessels), and oxidation of plasma lipoprotein (lipid bound to protein). These forms of smoking-induced damage can also amplify the risk of heart disease.

Tobacco smoking induces inflammatory reactions. The products of inflammatory reactions, such as free radicals, pro-inflammatory cytokines, complement proteins (which are toxic to cells), adhesion molecules, and prostaglandins (a product of fatty acids) are released in excessive amounts, which can increase the risk of cancer. Tobacco smoking also causes damage to genetic material, which can increase the risk of cancer. Tobacco smoking lowers the levels of certain antioxidants (vitamins A and C and beta-carotene), and B vitamins (cyanocobalamin and folic acid). The concentration of vitamin C declines in the breast milk of female smokers, and this can increase oxidative stress in breast-feeding children.

The red blood cells of smokers are more susceptible to lipid peroxidation (membrane damage) than those of nonsmokers. Supplementation with vitamin E has been reported to limit lipid peroxidation produced by free radicals. Smoking also results in folic acid deficiency, primarily affecting bronchial epithelial (lung) cells, which become abnormal—a process called metaplasia. This abnormality can lead to dysplasia, a precursor to cancer. Supplementation with 10 milligrams of folate and 0.5 milligram of vitamin B_{12} helps curb the above abnormality in the lungs. At present there are no recommendations for how to reduce the risk of cancer in tobacco smokers, except for recommending they quit smoking. For those who are in the process of quitting or who are unable to quit because of severe addiction, we suggest that the diet and lifestyle modifications, and micronutrient supplementation, recommended in this book for cancer prevention may reduce tobacco smoking–related cancer risk. Such a strategy may also reduce the risk of other adverse health effects related to smoking, such as heart disease.

What is the risk of cancer among nonsmokers who are exposed to tobacco smoke? Some human survey–type studies suggest that there is a significant increase in lung cancer risk among nonsmoking spouses of smokers—about two times higher than that found among nonsmoking couples. Thus, passive smoke inhalation (secondhand smoke) also increases the risk of some cancers. A few epidemiologic studies have revealed that both active and passive tobacco smoking are associated with increased risk of breast cancer, renal carcinoma, and bladder cancer (Johnson 2005; Kropp and Chang-Claude 2008; Hemelt et al. 2009). However, other, similar types of studies with specific cancers produced inconsistent results. Lifetime exposure to active or passive tobacco smoking was not associated with alterations in breast cancer, esophageal cancer, or gastric adenocarcinoma. Despite some conflicting results, cessation of active and passive tobacco smoking must be included in a cancer-prevention strategy. Smoking can also cause birth defects in fetuses. The children of smoking parents (one or both parents) may have a higher risk of lung cancer. For these reasons nonsmokers should avoid surroundings with high amounts of tobacco smoke. It is encouraging that smoking is now prohibited in most public and many private places around the United States, a policy that is being adopted by many other countries around the world.

The public and private programs that aim to prevent smoking should be pursued vigorously. Efforts must be made to encourage those who are addicted to tobacco smoking or chewing to quit. In addition, we suggest that the diet and lifestyle modifications, and micronutrient supplementation, recommended in this book for cancer prevention may reduce tobacco smoking–related cancer and other risks.

The Use of Cell Phones

Cell-phone technology and its use have exploded during the past decade throughout the world. About five billion people use cell phones at this time, and this number is likely to continue to grow. The fact that radio-frequency electromagnetic radiation, a form of non-ionizing radiation, from cell phones can be absorbed into the brain has prompted concerns that regular cell-phone use for a long period of time may increase the risk of acoustic neuroma (a benign brain tumor) and other brain tumors. The effects of cell-phone use on cancer risk have been investigated using primarily epidemiologic methodologies. The results of these studies have been inconsistent, varying from no effect to adverse effects (Han et al. 2009; Kan et al. 2008; Hardell and Sage 2008). Reviews of several studies on the effect of cell-phone use on the risk of brain tumors revealed that regular use of cell phones for a period of ten years or more was associated with increased risk of acoustic neuroma and glioma (a deadly form of brain tumor) (Hardell et al. 2007; Hardell et al. 2008). Other epidemiologic studies reported no such association between cell-phone use and risk of brain tumor (Takebayashi et al. 2006; Croft et al. 2008). In another epidemiologic study, regular use of cell phones was associated with increased risk of benign parotid (salivary) gland tumors

(Sadetzki 2008). An epidemiologic study on an Egyptian population living near a cell-phone base station revealed that these people were at increased risk of developing neuropsychiatric problems, such as headache, memory changes, dizziness, tremors, depressive symptoms, and sleep disturbances, compared to a control population not living near the base (Abdel-Rassoul 2007). This observation has not been confirmed in another population.

Laboratory studies on the effect of cell phones on cancer risk in animals and cell culture are very few. The radio-frequency radiation emitted from a cell phone produced no effect on cancer incidence in mice (Tillmann et al. 2007). Exposure of mammalian cells in culture to an 835-MHz radio-frequency radiation electromagnetic field slightly enhanced the levels of chemical-induced genetic damage (Kim et al. 2008).

Epidemiologic studies reveal an association between cell-phone use and cancer risk. (Epidemiologic studies do not suggest a direct cause-effect relationship.) These studies are not sufficient to conclude that cell phone use directly increases the risk of brain cancer. From the epidemiologic studies it is not possible to conclude that a particular agent is cancer causing or cancer protective. A causal relationship can only be established if a clinical study in which an intervening agent (cell-phone use) is administered for a specific time period, and the clinical end point—such as risk of cancer—is determined at the end of the study period. Because of the long latent period between continuous exposures to radio-frequency electromagnetic radiation from a cell phone and the development of adverse effects, and because of the radiation's potential interaction with other agents during this period, conclusive data from epidemiologic studies alone are difficult to obtain. More studies need to be done.

The current controversies regarding the effects of cell-phone use on cancer risk are analogous to those encountered on the carcinogenic potential of low doses of ionizing radiation. For decades many people denied that low-dose ionizing radiation was carcinogenic; only recently has it been accepted as a human carcinogen by federal agencies. We hope that the controversy surrounding the effects of cell-phone use on human health will be settled sooner, because of its potential health implications around the world. At this time it is prudent to avoid excessive and unnecessary use of cell phones. In addition, we suggest that the diet and lifestyle modifications, and micronutrient supplementation, recommended in this book for cancer prevention may reduce any possible cell-phone-related cancer risk.

EXAMPLES OF DIET-RELATED CANCER-CAUSING SUBSTANCES

Human diets contain both cancer-protective and cancer-causing substances (Ames 1983). Most of the mutagenic and carcinogenic substances that are present in the diet are naturally occurring; however, small amounts of mutagens have been introduced into the diet by the use of pesticides in agriculture. The relative ratio of protective and mutagenic substances in a human diet can vary markedly from one individual to another and from one day to another in the same individual. Varying levels of mutagens and carcinogens are formed during storage of food at room temperature and during the cooking process. For example, flame-broiled fatty meat may contain much higher levels of carcinogens like benzo(a)pyrene than grilled meat. Consumption of a nitrite-rich diet (bacon, sausage, cured meat) can form nitrosamine in the stomach at an acid pH through the combination of nitrites and secondary amines. Diets rich in meat increase the levels of mutagens in the feces compared to vegetarian diets. Consumption of highly caloric diets and diets rich in fat can also increase the risk of cancer. Epidemiologic studies have reported that the acrylamide that is formed during the heating of several foods at very high temperature is associated with the increased risk of endometrial, ovarian, estrogen-positive breast cancer, and renal cancer in women but not with lung cancer in men. It is also associated with a decreased risk of lung cancer in women (Hogervorst et al. 2009). Aflatoxin alone or in combination with hepatitis B virus can increase the risk of liver cancer (Wogan et al. 2004).

Food Storage

Potential cancer-causing substances can form during the storage of food at room temperature. The browning of vegetables or fruits at room temperature is an indication of the formation of mutagenic substances such as oxidized phenolic compound, which have been damaged by oxygen. This form of phenolic compounds can in turn damage genetic material in the cells. Normally, phenolic compounds present in the fruits and vegetables act as powerful antioxidants. Hydrazine (a reducing agent chemical) is often sprayed in very small amounts over salads and vegetables to prevent oxidation and keep them fresh for a longer period of time. Hydrazine can also cause an allergic reaction in some people.

Cooking

Cooking at high temperatures can cause excessive browning of meats and vegetables. This is an indication of the formation of mutagenic substances that can damage DNA. Although foods prepared in such a manner are considered tasty, their consumption should be avoided or at least reduced.

What happens when meat is cooked over charcoal? Cooking meat over charcoal is an extremely popular practice in the United States. Studies suggest that this practice, if done frequently, may increase the risk of cancer. If it is done in moderation and in combination with the steps recommended in this book for cancer prevention, cancer risk may be reduced considerably. To understand this, let us examine what happens when meat is cooked over heated charcoal.

As the meat cooks, fat drips down onto the hot charcoal, generating smoke that contains polycyclic aromatic hydrocarbons such as benzo(a)pyrene, a powerful cancer-causing agent. The cooking meat absorbs the smoke. Thus, charcoal-broiled meat contains cancer-causing substances from the smoke, whereas meat that is not charcoal-broiled does not. The amount of polycyclic aromatic hydrocarbons increases if the fat content of the meat is high and if it is cooked under conditions that expose it to high levels of fat-generated smoke. The average charcoal-broiled steak can contain about 8 micrograms of polycyclic aromatic hydrocarbons per kilogram of steak.

In order to minimize the amounts of cancer-causing substances in charcoal-broiled meat, it is important to remove as much fat as possible from the meat before cooking. In addition, the meat should be placed a little farther away from the charcoal during cooking so that at least some of the fat-generated smoke will dissipate into the air before it reaches the meat. Covering the grill during cooking may be harmful, because all smoke will be absorbed by the meat. The cook and others should avoid inhaling the smoke. Alternatively, propane-powered grills can be used, so that people can still enjoy a barbecue without magnifying their exposure to potential cancer-causing agents.

Digestion

Mutagens and carcinogens are formed during digestion. Nitrites typically are used to preserve meat and are present in bacon, sausage, hot dogs, and cured meat. Meat without nitrites can easily be infected with harmful microorganisms that can cause severe sickness and even death in some cases. Nitrites by themselves do not cause cancer, but they can combine with amines in the stomach to form nitrosamines. Nitrosamines are among the most potent cancer-causing agents for both animals and human beings. They are soluble in water and therefore can be absorbed readily and distributed to all tissues of the body. The presence of antioxidants, such as vitamin C or E (d-alpha-tocopherol) in the stomach may prevent the formation of or lower the levels of nitrosamines.

Thus, taking vitamin C or E before eating food containing nitrites may limit or prevent the formation of nitrosamines in the stomach. The necessary amount of either vitamin depends on the amount of nitrites consumed. At this time, the precise amount of these vitamins has not been determined, but the micronutrients proposed in this book for cancer prevention should be sufficient to block the formation of cancer-causing agents from nitrites. In addition to nitrosamines, many other mutagenic substances are formed in the intestinal tract; not all of these lead to cancer formation, but some do.

Studies have shown that the levels of mutagenic substances in the feces are higher in people who are meat eaters than in those who are vegetarians (Reddy, Sharma, and Wynder 1980; Hayatsu, Hayatsu, and Wataya 1986). Higher levels of fecal mutagenic substances may increase the risk of cancer. This hypothesis is supported by the fact that the incidence of cancer among Seventh Day Adventists, a religious group in the United States who are vegetarians, is much lower than those who eat meat (Wynder, Lemon, and Bross 1959). Another study has reported that taking vitamin C or E (400 milligrams) reduces the levels of mutagenic substances in the feces of meat eaters (Dion et al. 1982). Furthermore, reports indicate that taking both vitamins is more effective than taking either individually. Therefore, an appropriate preparation of multiple vitamins, such as the ones we recommended in this book, may curb the formation of mutagenic and carcinogenic agents in the gastrointestinal tract.

Excessive Fat

The average American diet contains about 34.1 percent of calories from fat. Animal experiments (Reddy 1993) and human epidemiologic studies (Giovannucci et al. 1994) have revealed that this level of fat consumption may increase the risk of certain types of cancer, particularly breast, colon, prostate, and possibly other cancers. Conversely, reducing fat intake lessens the risk of these cancers. High levels of fat, therefore, act as a tumor promoter. There is no exact explanation for the effects of a high-fat diet on increasing cancer risk, but some laboratory studies have reported that the production of prostaglandin E_2 (PGE_2), a chemical that is produced by lipids in the body, is greatly increased in animals that are fed a high-fat diet (Rao and Reddy 1993). High levels of PGE_2 have been shown to impair the body's immune system. Therefore, the amplified cancer risk brought about by a high-fat diet may be due to the suppression of the body's defense system against cancer. High doses of vitamin E succinate may block some of the harmful effects of excessive fat consumption by reducing the action of PGE_2 on cells (Prasad, Cole, and Hovland 1998). This does not mean that one should continue eating a high-fat diet and take large amounts of vitamin E; a high-fat diet may still heighten the risk of heart attack. The relationship between diet- and lifestyle-related agents and cancer risk is listed in Table 4.1.

TABLE 4.1. PROBABLE DIETARY- AND LIFESTYLE-RELATED CAUSATIVE AGENTS AND INCREASED RISK OF CANCER

Causative agents	Type of cancer
Excessive fat	Prostate, breast, stomach, colon, rectum, pancreas, kidney
Excess protein	Breast, endometrium, prostate, colon, rectum, pancreas, kidney
Excess total calories	Most cancers
Alcohol	Esophagus, mouth, head, neck, lip, stomach, liver, colon, breast, rectum
Tobacco smoking	Lung, cervix, larynx, mouth, esophagus
Excess caffeine/coffee	Pancreas, lung, liver, mouth, larynx, bladder
Excess saccharine	Bladder
Cadmium from diet or smoking	Kidney
Excess zinc	All cancers, especially breast and stomach
Iron deficiency	Stomach and esophagus
Iodine deficiency	Thyroid
Excess smoked meat or fish	Stomach
Charcoal-broiled meat; pickled products	Stomach
Cancer-causing viruses	Liver, certain blood cancers, cervix

From K. N. Prasad and K. C. Prasad, *Fight Cancer with Vitamins and Supplements*, Rochester, Vt.: Healing Arts Press, 2001.

A high-fat diet can raise the levels of circulating estrogen in females (Adlercreutz et al. 1994), and high levels of estrogen are known to act as a tumor promoter. In addition, the presence of large amounts of bile acids and fatty acids from a diet rich in fat may promote colon cancer, because these substances encourage the proliferation of cells in the colon. Increased cell proliferation makes colon cells more sensitive to cancer formation. Dietary calcium inhibits this action of bile acids and fatty acids by making them insoluble and rendering them unavailable for absorption. Our proposed micronutrient preparation for cancer prevention can also help prevent increased proliferation of cells.

Excess Protein

Limited laboratory data and human studies suggest that excessive consumption of protein may be associated with a higher risk of cancer of the breast, endometrium, prostate, colon, rectum, pancreas, and kidney. Lower protein intake seems to reduce the risk of these cancers. Although animal studies suggest that excess protein has a specific role in animal cancer, human studies are not persuasive. Since the Western diet contains significant amounts of meat, which is a rich source of both protein and fat, it is difficult to determine the independent role of protein in human cancer formation. Animal experiments show that a high protein intake increases the incidence of chemically induced tumors, which may indicate that proteins have a similar role in human cancer. Additional studies are needed. We suggest avoiding excessive consumption of proteins.

Excess Total Calories and Carbohydrates

Limited animal and human studies suggest that excessive total calories may increase the risk of cancer in humans by acting as a tumor promoter. There are no scientific data to suggest that an excessive intake of carbohydrates is directly related to the increased risk of cancer in animals or humans; however, excessive consumption of carbohydrates may increase total caloric intake. Additional studies are needed to define the role of excess calories and carbohydrates in human carcinogenesis.

EXAMPLES OF DIET-RELATED
CANCER PROTECTIVE AGENTS

Antioxidants

Protective substances in the diet include antioxidants. The levels and types of antioxidant can vary widely depending on the type of food. Generally, fruits and green, red, or yellow vegetables are rich in antioxidants. Consumption of meat or fish provides endogenous antioxidants that may decrease as a function of aging. Lower intake of nutrients, especially antioxidants, from the diet can increase the risk of cancer.

In addition to standard dietary antioxidants such as vitamins A, C, and E and carotenoids and selenium, there are several other antioxidants, including many polyphenolic compounds present in fruits, vegetables, and herbs and that exhibit properties that are relevant to cancer prevention. These polyphenols are a group of chemical substances found in plants, which are also referred to as phytochemicals. They include tannins, lignins, and flavonoids. The largest and best-studied polyphenols are flavonoids, which include quercetin, epicatechin, and oligomeric proanthocyanidins. The major sources of flavonoids include all citrus fruits, berries, ginkgo biloba, onions, parsley, tea, red wine, and dark chocolate. Resveratrol, a flavonoid that has drawn a great deal of attention in recent years, is found in grape skin and grape seed. More than five thousand naturally occurring flavonoids have been characterized from various plants. Flavonoids are poorly absorbed by the intestinal tract in humans, but all possess varying degrees of antioxidant activity. These polyphenolic compounds do not exhibit any unique function in cancer prevention that cannot be produced by standard dietary (vitamins A, C, and E and carotenoids and selenium) and endogenous (alpha-lipoic acid, L-carnitine, n-acetylcysteine, and coenzyme Q10) antioxidants. Therefore, their inclusion in the proposed multiple-micronutrient preparation for cancer prevention may not be necessary.

Dietary Fiber

The reference for this section has been provided in a review (Prasad, Cole, and Hovland 1998). Human and animal studies suggest that a diet containing high levels of fiber may lower the risk of certain cancers, especially colon cancer. The incidence of colon cancer is very small among people of northwest India (in the state of Punjab), who eat a diet rich in roughage, cellulose, vegetables, fiber, and yogurt, compared with southern Indians, who eat less fiber. As noted previously, the incidence of cancer is much lower among Seventh Day Adventists, who are vegetarians.

A diet rich in fiber results in regular bowel movements, which minimize the body's contact time with cancer-causing substances normally formed in the intestinal tract and thus reduces the risk of cancer. Higher amounts of fiber bind increased amounts of intestinal cholesterol, bile acids, and mutagens and carcinogens that are formed during digestion and eliminate them in the feces. This reduces intestinal absorption and exposure time of the intestinal cells to these potentially carcinogenic substances. Therefore, studies have assumed that only cancer of the intestinal tract would be reduced by fiber's mechanism of action. However, high fiber consumption also reduces the recurrence of breast cancer, which suggests that additional mechanisms of cancer protection from high fiber may exist. Indeed, it has been reported that, with the help of endogenous bacteria that are present in the colon, high fiber intake can generate millimolar (very high) levels of butyric acid, a small, 4-carbon fatty acid that is absorbed rapidly. Several studies have reported that butyrate and its analog, phenyl butyrate, have exhibited strong effects against tumors other than intestinal-tract cancer. Thus, a high-fiber diet may provide protection not only against colon cancer but also against other tumors. Following a low-fat and high-fiber diet is essential for the proposed cancer-prevention strategy.

THE IMPACT OF THE DIFFERENCES IN THE ANIMAL DIET AND THE HUMAN DIET ON CANCER-PREVENTION STUDIES IN HUMANS

Studies on the effect of micronutrients on cancer prevention are generally performed on animals, the results of these studies are taken into consideration when scientists design human studies. In contrast to human diets in the United States, the laboratory rodent's diet is vegetarian and relatively uniform in content. Therefore, the ratio of protective and carcinogenic substances in this animal's diet may not vary significantly during the study period. As stated previously, human diets can vary markedly from day to day and within one individual in the amounts of cancer-protective and cancer-causing substances. In addition, most rodents (except guinea pigs) make their own vitamin C; however, humans do not. There may be differences in the metabolism of cancer-causing substances and cancer-protective substances between animals and humans. These and other differences have convinced us that the results of studies featuring micronutrients in cancer prevention in animals should not be extrapolated to the design of human studies with respect to number, type, dose, and dose schedule of antioxidants.

CONCLUDING REMARKS

Many human cancers are associated with environmental, dietary, and lifestyle-related mutagens and carcinogens. The risk of many cancers can be reduced if we avoid exposure to these substances. Individuals cannot control the levels of mutagens and carcinogens present in the environment (air and water); this requires federal regulation, which is not easily accomplished. We can, however, control the diet- and lifestyle-related factors that are known to increase the risk of cancer. In addition, we suggest that micronutrient supplementation may reduce the risk of spontaneous cancers as well as those induced by mutagens and carcinogens associated with environment, diet, and lifestyle.

5 Diagnostic Doses of Radiation and Cancer

Diagnostic radiation procedures are primarily low-dose X-rays or gamma rays, also known as ionizing radiation, that allow detection of certain abnormalities in the body. Ionizing radiation is very harmful and can induce somatic mutations (genetic changes during one's lifetime) and heritable mutations (genetic changes that are transmitted to future generations). Although X-rays and gamma rays can cause cancer and certain noncancerous diseases, they are very useful in the diagnosis of human diseases as well as in the treatment of cancer. Children are more vulnerable to radiation-induced damage than adults. Also, when children are exposed to diagnostic doses of radiation they are at greater risk than adults for developing some of the harmful effects of radiation that can take many years to manifest.

During the past two decades the growing use of X-ray-based devices has raised concerns about the potential of such procedures for increasing the risk of cancer and somatic and heritable mutations. These risks also exist in radiation workers. As previously noted, radiation workers include those who work with radiation equipment, those who work at nuclear power plants, and the pilots and crews of civilian and military aircrafts who are exposed to higher doses of cosmic radiation per year than non-radiation workers. The number of radiation workers has increased proportionally with the increased number of diagnostic radiation procedures. In 2008, more than sixty million computed tomography

(CT) scans were performed in the United States (Shah and Platt 2008). This number does not include other diagnostic procedures such as chest X-rays, dental X-rays, fluoroscopic imaging, positron emission tomography (PET), and other nuclear-medicine scans. Cardiologists alone prescribe and/or directly perform more than 50 percent of radiation-imaging examinations, which contribute to about two-thirds of the total effective radiation dose to patients. About twenty million nuclear-medicine examinations were performed in 2006, and cardiac examinations accounted for about 57 percent of all nuclear-medicine procedures and 85 percent of the radiation dose (Amis et al. 2007). Therefore, it is likely that many more patients were exposed to diagnostic doses of radiation than estimated. About five billion imaging examinations are performed worldwide each year, and two out of three involve ionizing radiation.

In addition to patients who undergo diagnostic radiation procedures and radiation workers, frequent flyers receive higher doses of radiation than those who fly infrequently, because of the increased exposure to cosmic radiation that occurs during air travel. These individuals are potentially at higher risk of developing cancer. Some human epidemiologic studies have suggested that long-term use of cell phones can increase the risk of brain cancer, although this has not been established by laboratory experiments (Han et al. 2009; Kan et al. 2008; Hardell and Sage 2008). Nevertheless, we have to be concerned about the potential risk of excessive cell-phone use. Because of the potential health hazards of low doses of radiation, developing an effective radiation-protection strategy that involves both radiation-dose reduction and tissue-protection methods has become an urgent issue.

HOW DOES RADIATION CONVERT NORMAL CELLS TO CANCER CELLS?

Radiation-induced cancer is no different from cancer that occurs spontaneously or that is caused by other tumor-causing agents (tumor initiators/tumor promoters). Initially, radiation causes mutations in normal dividing cells. These mutated cells gradually accumulate additional mutations from exposure to various cancer-causing substances and increased radiation doses. The mutations continue to occur over a long period of time, and eventually convert the mutated cells into cancer cells. Radiation-induced human cancers have long latent periods; for example, the latent period for leukemia is up to ten years, while lung and breast tumors may take thirty years or more to develop. This suggests that radiation-induced mutations (some of which can be detected within twenty-four hours after radiation exposure) are not directly responsible for the conversion of normal human cells to cancer cells, because such cells continue to divide, differentiate, and die like non-irradiated normal cells for a long period of time. However, radiation-induced mutations cause genetic instability in normal cells that can make these cells more vulnerable to additional genetic changes that continue to occur over a long period of time. Eventually, a defect in expression of maturation (differentiation) genes prevents mutated cells from going through the natural cell cycle that culminates in cell death. These abnormal, "immortal" cells continue to divide in an uncontrolled manner, the first step in cancer formation.

Immortalized cells can continue to proliferate and can form a mass, such as polyps in the colon. When some key cellular genes, such as oncogenes (cancer-causing genes) or tumor-suppressor genes, are changed by continued exposure to radiation or tumor-causing substances, the cells can then become cancerous. The long latent period for radiation-induced cancer provides an opportunity for medical intervention at any time after radiation exposure with the appropriate radioprotective agents, in order to reduce the risk of late-forming adverse effects.

X-rays cause damage to cells primarily by producing excessive amounts of free radicals with very little damage from the direct effect of radiation, which is also called ionization. Free radicals that are generated from cancer-causing substances in the environment, diet, and lifestyle continue to change genetic activity in the irradiated cells. Therefore, it appears rational to suggest that supplementation with antioxidants that are known to neutralize free radicals, before radiation exposure or any time after irradiation, may reduce the risk of developing cancer.

Unit of Radiation Dose

The current dosage unit of X-rays or gamma rays is Gy (named after famous radiobiologist Dr. L. Harold Gray), which refers to a dose that is absorbed in the tissue. One Gy equals 100 rad (radiation absorbed dose). Some types of radiation, such as proton or neutron radiation, at the same dose of Gy are more effective than X-rays or gamma rays. In order to account for this difference in effects, the unit of radiation dose is expressed as Sv (named after famous health physicist Dr. Rolf Sievert), which is used in radiation-protection recommendations. One Sv equals 100 rem (roentogen equivalent man).

Radiation doses delivered during various diagnostic procedures are listed in Tables 4 to 6. One Sv equals 1,000 mSv; 1 mSv (milliSv) equals 100 mrem. Radiation dose is frequently expressed in mSv. For X-rays and gamma rays, 1 Gy equals about 1 Sv.

TABLE 5.1. SUMMARY OF ESTIMATED EFFECTIVE RADIATION DOSE FROM COMMON DIAGNOSTIC PROCEDURES

Type of examination	Effective dose (mSV)
Standard radiography	0.01–10.0
Computed tomography	2.0–20.0
Nuclear medicine	0.3–20.0
Interventional procedure	5.0–70.0

From K. N. Prasad, *Micronutrients in Health and Disease,* Boca Raton, Fla.: Francis and Taylor Publishing Groups, 2011.

TABLE 5.2. ESTIMATED DOSES OF IONIZING RADIATION DELIVERED DURING SPECIFIC DIAGNOSTIC PROCEDURES

Procedure type	Effective dose (mSv)
Chest or dental X-ray	0.01
Electron-beam CT (cardiac)	1.0–1.3
Electron-beam CT coronary angiography	1.5–2.0
Catheter coronary angiography	2.1–2.5
Electron-beam CT whole body	5.2
CT (head)	2.0
CT (abdomen)	10.0
Barium enema	7.0
Upper GI exam	3.0
IV urogram	2.5
Lumbar spine	1.3
Mammogram	7.0
Passenger from Athens to New York	0.06
Occupational annual dose limit	50.0*
General public annual dose limit	1.0
Background annual dose at sea level	1.0

*Occupational and general public dose limit does not include background radiation.
From K. N. Prasad, *Micronutrients in Health and Disease,* Boca Raton, Fla.: Francis and Taylor Publishing Groups, 2011.

TABLE 5.3. ESTIMATED DOSES OF RADIATION FROM SELECTED RADIOACTIVE ISOTOPE ADMINISTERED ONCE DURING NUCLEAR-MEDICINE PROCEDURES

Procedure type	Effective dose (mSv)
18F-Flurodeoxyglucose	10 mCi 4.8
99mTc-MAA lung scan	5 mCi 0.60
99mTc-HDP bone scan	20 mCi 4.0
201Tl Thallium scan	3 mCi 0.60

From K. N. Prasad, *Micronutrients in Health and Disease,* Boca Raton, Fla.: Francis and Taylor Publishing Groups, 2011.

Radiation Enhances the Effect of Cancer-Causing Substances in the Environment

The important consequences of radiation interacting with other cancer-causing substances are often ignored by many radiologists and radiation scientists while evaluating the risk of diagnostic doses of radiation. Laboratory experiments have shown that radiation can enhance the effect of cancer-causing chemicals and viruses, resulting in an increased incidence of cancer. Some examples are given below. In laboratory experiments on normal cells, X-rays enhanced the incidence of chemical-induced cancer by about ninefold (DiPaolo, Donavan, and Popewscu 1976) and ultraviolet radiation–induced cancer by about twelvefold (Judy, W. V., Folkers, K., and Hall 1991). X-rays also enhanced the level of ozone- and viral-induced cancer by about two- to threefold (Pollock and Todaro 1968; Borek et al. 1986). Radiation doses that alone do not convert normal cells to cancer cells do so when combined with a tumor promoter. Ionizing radiation in combination with tobacco smoking increases the risk of lung cancer by about 50 percent. A low dose of radiation (20 mSV) does not produce detectable levels of genetic damage; however, in the presence of caffeine (which inhibits the repair of DNA damage), genetic damage becomes detectable (Puck et al. 1993). Low doses of radiation (20 and 50 mSV) can enhance the rate of proliferation of normal cells (Suzuki, Kodama, and Watanabe 2001), a risk factor for development of cancer. Furthermore, lower doses (about 1 mSv) of radiation do not activate the repair system in the cells (Rothkamm and Lobrich 2003). This lack of repair after exposure to low doses of radiation can lead to accumulation of mutations, which in turn can increase the risk of cancer.

What Are Risk Estimates of Diagnostic Radiation–Induced Cancer in Humans?

Recent human studies have revealed that increased risk of cancer exists after exposure to diagnostic doses of radiation (Brenner and Sachs 2006; BEIR VII, Phase 2, 2006) although most practicing and academic radiologists and dentists downplay this risk of radiation. It should be remembered that during the 1960s some prominent scientists representing the tobacco industry denied that nicotine was an addictive substance and that tobacco smoking could increase the risk of cancer. It took more than a decade before these facts were accepted by all.

Most radiation scientists agree that cancer risk in humans following exposure to low doses of radiation may best be estimated by a linear no-threshold relationship in which any radiation dose has the potential to induce cancer. The most recent Biological Effects of Ionizing Radiation (BEIR VII) report, supported by an authoritative group of radiation scientists, agrees with this view of radiation-induced cancer formation. This idea of risk estimation for radiation-induced cancer can also be applied to children. The effective radiation dose estimates from some diagnostic procedures are presented in Tables 5.1 to 5.3. Estimates of cancer risks are presented in Table 5.4.

TABLE 5.4. ESTIMATED INCREASES IN CANCER RISK FROM EXPOSURE TO ONE COMPUTED TOMOGRAPHY (CT) SCAN

Source and dose of radiation	Increase in cancer risk in exposed individuals
Dose from one CT scan	1 per 1,000
Dose from one CT scan	1 per 1,200
Dose from one CT scan	2.9 per 1,000
Dose from one CT scan	0.26 per 1,000 females
Dose from one CT scan	0.2 per 1,000 males
15 mSv	1 per 750
20 mSV	1 per 500
25 mSv	1 per 400

The estimation of cancer risk from one CT scan in various studies varies from 0.2 per 1,000 to 2.9 per 1,000.

From K. N. Prasad, *Micronutrients in Health and Disease,* Boca Raton, Fla.: Francis and Taylor Publishing Groups, 2011.

CT Scans: The typical radiation dose for an adult from a chest CT scan can range between 6 to 10 mSv. The average annual dose from background radiation in the United States has increased from 1 mSv to approximately 3 mSv. Several radiation-dose estimates for imaging studies in adults and children have been published (Robbins 2008; Hal and Garcia 2006). A dose of radiation from a CT scan may increase the risk of cancer in children by 1 case in 1,000 exposed individuals (Rice et al. 2007; Hall 2002; Brenner et al. 2001) (see Table 7). The BEIR VII report has estimated that a dose of 15 mSv may increase cancer risk by 1 case in 750 (see Table 7). Others have estimated that coronary multislice computed tomography (MSCT) that delivers about 20 mSv may increase the risk of cancer by 1 case in 500 (BEIR VII 2006). A coronary stent procedure may increase the risk of cancer by 1 case in 400 for 25 mSv. If one considers the fact that children may be exposed to cancer-causing chemical and biological agents that increase radiation-induced cancer risk over a longer period of time, the estimates of cancer-mortality risk for children could be higher.

Another study has reported that the lifetime cancer-mortality risk for a one-year-old child exposed to radiation from a CT scan is 0.18 percent for an abdominal CT and 0.07 percent for a head CT. This risk is higher than for adults. In 2001 approximately 600,000 abdominal and head CT scans were performed on children under the age of fifteen years old, with the potential for up to five hundred of the exposed children to die from cancer attributed in part to CT radiation (Brenner et al. 2001). A Canadian study reported that an abdominal CT study in a five-year-old child may increase the lifetime risk of radiation-induced cancer by approximately 26.1 cases per 100,000 in females and 20.4 cases per 100,000 in males (Wan et al. 2008). Another study performed in Israel has estimated an increase of about 0.29 percent in the total number of patients who are expected to die from cancer due to radiation procedures (Chodick et al. 2007). If one considers the fact that patients receiving diagnostic doses of radiation and radiation workers may also be exposed during their lifetimes to other cancer-causing chemicals and viruses that enhance radiation-induced cancer risk, these estimates of cancer-mortality risk could be even higher.

Cardiovascular imaging: Recently, dose estimates and cancer risk from cardiovascular imaging have been published. In 2006, the estimated medical radiation exposure dose in the United States had reached 3.2 mSv per year, which is more than six times higher than that estimated in 2004 (Berrington de Gonzalez and Darby 2004). The analysis of the annual number of diagnostic X-rays taken in United Kingdom and fourteen other developed countries revealed that the cumulative risk varied from 0.6 to 1.8 percent, whereas in Japan, which used the highest number of annual diagnostic X-rays, it was more than 3 percent (Berrington de Gonzalez and Darby 2004).

Pilots and Aircraft Crews: Military and civilian pilots and flight attendants of aircrafts are exposed to cosmic radiation, potential chemical carcinogens (fuel and jet engine exhaust), and electromagnetic fields from cockpit instruments and experience disrupted sleep patterns. Several epidemiologic studies have evaluated the risk of cancer in these populations. Most suggest that there is an increased risk of prostate cancer, melanoma and other skin cancer, and acute myeloid leukemia in male pilots and breast cancer, melanoma, and bone cancer in female flight attendants (Buja et al. 2005; Band et al. 1996; Sigurdson and Ron 2004; Rafnsson et al. 2001; Pukkala, Auvinen, and Wahlberg 1995).

Dental X-rays: Dental X-rays are essential for evaluating dental problems. But some studies have shown that soon after dental X-rays, the formation of micronuclei (the breaking of the cell's nucleus into very small pieces) in the cells of the oral cavity is induced in both adults and in children; other studies have disputed this finding (Cerqueira et al. 2008; Angelleri et al. 2007; Papova et al. 2007). The long-term significance of this is unknown; however, it is important to note that even very small doses of X-rays can cause measurable damage to cells soon after irradiation. Therefore, every effort should be made to provide tissue protection during dental X-rays, especially since the oral cavity cannot be protected by a lead apron. In addition, a lead collar should be placed around the neck in order to protect the thyroid gland.

An epidemiologic study published in the *Journal of Acta Oncologica* in 2010 by Dr. Anjum Memon of Brighton and Sussex Medical School in the United Kingdom and his collaborators at Cambridge University and Kuwait University revealed that the risk of thyroid cancer increased by about twofold in men and women who received four dental X-rays, by about fourfold in those who received five to nine dental X-rays, and more than fivefold in those who received ten or more dental X-rays. The British Dental Association spokesperson has questioned these results.

Medical organizations have often questioned observations that challenge their current viewpoint. For example, the cure for scurvy remained limited to the Native American Indians for almost two hundred years because of the stubborn position of the medical establishment in France. (See page 35 for more on this topic.)

What Are the Types of Radiation-Induced Non-Cancerous Diseases?

The incidence of non-cancerous diseases, such as thyroid-gland enlargement and dry-eye syndrome, can increase after exposure to low doses of radiation. This was investigated in children living in radiation-contaminated areas near the Chernobyl nuclear accident site in the Ukraine. The accident occurred on April 26, 1986. The incidence of thyroid-gland enlargement and vision disorders (mostly dry-eye syndrome) was closely related to the levels of radiation released from the radioactive contaminated area (Ben-Amotz et al. 1998). Increased levels of markers of free-radical damage were also found among these children (Korkina, Afanas'ef, and Diplock 1993).

Current Controversies Surrounding Mammograms

Mammography is an X-ray-based procedure that can detect breast cancer at an early stage, but about one-third of the women screened have false-positive results, requiring additional evaluations (biopsies of the breast tissue; additional imaging tests) even though no breast cancer is found. In addition, the false-positive results create anxiety that could cause psychological harm. Some studies have estimated that mammography reduces breast-cancer mortality by 1 case in 2,000 screened women; the other 1,999 women do not benefit. The current recommendation for mammography is one per year for women forty or older.

Other imaging procedures for detecting breast cancer include MRI (magnetic resonance imaging) and ultrasound, which do not emit ionizing radiation–like X-rays. These modalities could be useful for screening purposes.

In the November 2009 the U.S. Preventive Services Task Force made new recommendations. They are:

1. Biennial mammography for women aged fifty to seventy-four years.
2. The decision to start regular, biennial mammography before the age of fifty years should be left to the patient and should take into account her beliefs regarding specific benefits and harms.
3. The current evidence is insufficient to assess the additional benefits and harms of conducting mammography in women seventy-five years or older.
4. Do not teach breast self-examination.
5. The current evidence is insufficient to assess the additional benefits and harms of clinical breast examination beyond screening.
6. The current evidence is insufficient to assess the additional benefits and harms of either digital mammography or magnetic resonance imaging (MRI) instead of film mammography as screening modalities for breast cancer.

These recommendations generated a strong negative reaction from many radiologists as well as from the American Cancer Society and breast-cancer advocacy groups. However, some researchers and physicians defended the recommendations on the grounds that the cost of additional clinical evaluations (including discomfort and complications associated with biopsy) and their psychological harm outweigh a very small benefit on breast-cancer mortality reduction.

The potential risk of radiation from low-energy X-rays is about four times more damaging than high-energy X-rays for the same dose of radiation. In the discussion of the pros and cons of mammography, this finding was mostly ignored. We believe that this is an important risk factor that should be discussed with patients under the age of fifty years before screening. The radiation dose delivered to breast tissue during mammography varies from about 2 mSv to 20 mSv per film. The radiation dose from one breast CT scan is about 5 to 6 mSv. Studies have suggested that one CT scan can increase the risk of cancer by about one case per one thousand individuals. This risk is greater than the benefits produced by mammography (reduction in breast-cancer mortality by one case per two thousand screened women). It is also important to explore the screening value of other imaging techniques such as ultrasound and MRI, which do not produce X-rays. Whenever it is necessary to undergo mammography, efforts should be made to provide sufficient amounts of antioxidants that can reduce the potential risk of radiation.

Current Recommended Methods of Reducing Radiation Doses

An effective radiation-protection strategy should be based on methods for reducing radiation doses as much as possible without sacrificing the quality of the image. A radiation-protection strategy should also be based on tissue protection against radiation damage. Efforts to develop protection against radiation damage began soon after the discovery of X-rays in 1895 by Dr. Wilhelm Röntgen, a German scientist. However, the observation by Dr. H. J. Muller of Columbia University in the United States in 1927 that X-rays cause gene mutations in *Drosophila melanogaster* (common fruit fly) provided new motivation for the development of an effective protection strategy against radiation damage. The initial recommendations for radiation protection involved three principles that can reduce dose levels: (a) lead shielding of exposed areas, especially radiosensitive organs such as bone marrow, intestines, reproductive organs, and thyroid; (b) increased distance between the radiation source and radiation workers or patients; and (c) reduction of radiation exposure time. Each of these principles has been very useful in reducing dose levels during diagnostic radiation procedures, but they have a few important limitations, which are described below.

Limitations of Lead Shielding

During diagnostic radiation procedures, such as fluoroscopy, which delivers radiation to the small intestine, it may not be possible to protect the gastrointestinal tract (one of the organs most sensitive to radiation) with lead shielding. During this procedure, the skin cells are not protected from radiation damage. Shielding the body in areas away from the site of irradiation can protect radiosensitive organs such as the ovaries, testes, and skin cells. Radiologists who perform the above diagnostic procedures use lead aprons, but these do not protect skin cells of the arms or protect the eye (the lens is very sensitive to radiation damage). Many dentists provide lead aprons to patients to cover the lower portion of the body during dental X-ray; others do not. All patients undergoing any kind of diagnostic radiation procedure should demand lead aprons to cover at least the lower part of the body and the thyroid gland.

Limitations of Increasing the Distance
between Radiation Source and Recipient

Increasing the distance between the radiation source and the individual may not be practical for many radiation workers and patients. For radiation workers, this strategy may compromise patient care; in case of patients, it may reduce the quality of the image.

Limitations of Reducing
Radiation-Exposure Time

Reducing radiation-exposure time may also not be applicable to all populations, except those who are involved in taking care of patients who have received gamma-emitting radioactive isotope for medical purposes or who are responsible for radioactive decontamination as a result of nuclear accidents or attack.

ALARA (As Low as Reasonably Achievable)

To address the growing concerns of radiation-induced damage, additional recommendations have been made to reduce radiation doses in patients. These recommendations are called ALARA (as low as reasonably achievable), and they are supported by national and international radiation-protection agencies. At present, all radiologists and radiobiologists follow the principles of ALARA in order to reduce radiation doses to patients. Additional recommendations are also being made to reduce the number of diagnostic procedures in patients. These recommendations, no doubt, will be useful in reducing diagnostic radiation doses to patients; however, they do not provide any suggestions for how to provide protection to tissues in patients who receive low-dose radiation during diagnostic procedures. They also do not provide strategies for tissue protection among radiation workers who are exposed to radiation doses higher than non-radiation workers on a daily basis.

Proposed Methods of Tissue Protection

PAMARA
(Protection as Much as Reasonably Achievable)

The issue of protection of the tissues against the damage produced by diagnostic doses of radiation has not drawn adequate attention from radiation biologists or radiologists. At present, there is a lack of adequate tissue-protection strategy available for patients receiving diagnostic doses of radiation or for radiation workers. About 67 percent of radiation damage is caused by free radicals, which are produced during radiation exposure (Hall and Garcia 2006). Since antioxidants are known to neutralize free radicals and they have been shown to protect tissues against radiation damage, they may represent one of the best strategies for providing tissue protection against diagnostic doses of radiation. We have called this novel idea of tissue protection PAMARA (protection as much as reasonably achievable). Such a tissue-radiation protection strategy by antioxidants would be complementary to existing recommendations of dose reduction methods, including ALARA.

Tissue Radiation Protection, Including Cancer Risk Reduction, by Antioxidants

Several laboratory experiments and a few human studies have suggested that commonly used dietary and endogenous (made in the body) antioxidants that are nontoxic to humans can provide an effective radiation protection to tissue and cells. These antioxidants can also reduce the risk of cancer. The studies on radiation protection by the individual antioxidants are briefly described below.

Experiments Showing Tissue Protection by Antioxidants

Laboratory Experiments That Show Radiation Protection by Antioxidants

Twelve laboratory experiments with cells growing in petri dishes show that antioxidants protect against radiation-induced cancer formation and genetic damage. For example, vitamin E and selenium reduce radiation-induced cancer formation in vitro (Borek et al. 1986; Radner and Kennedy 1986). The combination of these two agents was more effective than the individual agents alone. Natural beta-carotene protected against radiation-induced cancer, whereas synthetic beta-carotene was ineffective in cell culture (Kennedy and Krinsky 1994). Vitamins E and C and beta-carotene reduced radiation-induced genetic damage (Gaziev et al. 1995; Konopacka, Widel, and Rzeszowska-Wolny 1998; Kumar et al. 2002; Ni and Pei 1997; O'Connor et al. 1977; Okunieff et al. 2008; Ushakova et al. 1999; Weiss and Landauer 2000; Weiss and Landauer 2003). These studies suggest that free radicals generated during radiation exposure can induce genetic damage that can be avoided by the use of antioxidants.

Thirteen laboratory experiments in animals have shown that antioxidants protect tissues against radiation damage when administered before radiation exposure. For example, alpha-lipoic acid, a glutathione-elevating agent made in the body, increased the survival rate of lethally irradiated animals by protecting bone marrow from radiation damage (Ramakrishnan, Wolfe, and Catravas 1992). Vitamin E, vitamin C, and beta-carotene protected the tissues of rats and mice against radiation damage (Okunieff et al. 2008; Weiss and Landauer 2000; Weiss and Landauer 2003; Blumenthal et al. 2000; El-Habit et al. 2000; Ershoff and Steers 1960; Harapanhalli et al. 1996; Mills 1988; Mutlu-Turkoglu et al. 2000; Narra et al. 1994; Umegaki et al. 1997). Vitamin A and beta-carotene protected normal tissue during radiation therapy in an animal model (Seifter, Padawar, and Levenson 1984). A combination of vitamins A, C, and E protected against radiation-induced damage to bone marrow during radiation therapy of cancer in animals (Blumenthal et al. 2000). Supplementation with L-selenomethionine and several different types of antioxidants (vitamin C, vitamin E, glutathione, n-acetylcysteine, alpha-lipoic acid, coenzyme Q10, and soybean-derived Bowman-Birk inhibitor) protected human and rat cells against radiation-induced free-radical damage (Guan et al. 2004; Kennedy et al. 2006; Wan et al. 2006).

All previous animal studies with individual antioxidants have utilized primarily the intraperitoneal (abdominal cavity) route of injection prior to radiation exposure. The oral administration of antioxidants before radiation exposure was ineffective in these studies. Therefore, the effectiveness of a commercially available multiple-antioxidant preparation containing dietary antioxidants (vitamins A, C, and E, and beta-carotene and selenium) and endogenous antioxidants (alpha-lipoic acid, N-acetylcysteine, and coenzyme Q10) in reducing radiation damage in animals was tested. In a pilot study we observed that this formulation of multiple antioxidants, when administered orally before radiation exposure, increased the survival rate of lethally irradiated mice from 0 to 40 percent. The same formulation of antioxidants, when administered orally before and after irradiation in sheep exposed to a very high dose of radiation (causing 100 percent death within seven days), increased the animals' survival time from seven days to thirty-eight days (Prasad and Jones, unpublished results at NASA at Houston).

Female fruit flies carrying a dominant mutation in the HOP (TUM-1) gene are considered at high risk for developing a leukemia-like tumor that is thought to be similar to the genetic basis of cancer in humans. Proton radiation markedly increased the levels of cancer in these fruit flies. The antioxidant formulation used in previous studies also blocked proton radiation–induced cancer in fruit flies (unpublished observation in collaboration with Dr. S. Bhattacharya of NASA, Moffett Field, Calif.). This observation of fruit flies is of particular interest, because, to our knowledge, this is the first demonstration in which the genetic basis of the disease can be prevented by antioxidants. Although the studies discussed above were performed with high radiation doses, free radicals are generated irrespective of dose levels, and the amounts of free radicals increase with the dose. These studies suggest that orally administered antioxidant treatment can provide tissue protection against radiation damage as well as reduce radiation-induced cancer formation.

Human Studies That Show
Radiation Protection by Antioxidants

Four human studies have showed that oral administration of antioxidants can provide tissue protection against radiation damage. For example, vitamin A and N-acetylcysteine (NAC) may be effective against radiation-induced cancer. Supplementation with alpha-lipoic acid for twenty-eight days lowered the levels of oxidative damage among children chronically exposed to low doses of radiation in the area radioactively contaminated by the Chernobyl nuclear accident (Ben-Amotz et al. 1998). In another study, beta-carotene supplementation reduced cellular damage in the same population of children (Korkina, Afanas'ef, and Diplock 1993). A combination of vitamin E and alpha-lipoic acid was more effective than the individual agents. These studies in humans are very exciting because they demonstrate that antioxidants can protect against the free-radical damage caused by low doses of radiation. Oral supplementation with beta-carotene also protected against radiation-induced mucositis (inflammation of the mucous membranes) during radiation therapy for cancer of the head and neck (Mills 1988).

Proposed Recommendations for
Radiation Protection in Humans

For optimal radiation protection, the following steps are recommended.

1. Follow all guidelines for reducing radiation dose levels during any diagnostic procedures.
2. Always ask for a lead apron to protect your body as much as possible before undergoing diagnostic radiation procedures.
3. Follow the recommendations for tissue-radiation protection that are described in the following section.

Recommended Antioxidants for
Tissue Protection during Diagnostic Radiation
Procedures and Frequent Flying in Aircraft

Based on the twenty-five laboratory and four human studies in which antioxidants have been shown to protect tissue and genetic material against radiation damage, we recommend a preparation of antioxidants, in one capsule, containing vitamin C, d-alpha-tocopheryl succinate, natural mixed carotenoids, and glutathione-elevating agents (n-acetyl-cysteine and alpha-lipoic acid), plus selenium. The antioxidant doses for children under the age of twelve years would be lower than adults. Patients receiving diagnostic doses of radiation would receive two capsules thirty to sixty minutes before and two capsules six to eight hours after a diagnostic radiation procedure. Those receiving a nuclear-medicine diagnostic procedure might receive two capsules before and two twice a day for three to five days after administration of a radioactive isotope, depending on the half-life of the isotope. Frequent flyers might take two capsules before boarding a flight and two capsules a few hours after arrival. This antioxidant preparation, BioShield R1, is available commercially.

Recommended Micronutrient Preparation for Tissue Protection in Radiation Workers and Aircraft Pilots and Attendants

Since radiation workers and pilots and crews of aircraft often work at least eight hours a day, five days a week, during their entire employment period, we recommend a separate micronutrient preparation that has not only dietary and endogenous antioxidants but also other micronutrients necessary for maintaining good health. This micronutrient preparation, BioShield R2, is commercially available and contains vitamin A, natural mixed carotenoids, vitamin C, d-alpha-tocopherol acetate, d-alpha-tocopheryl succinate, vitamin D, alpha-lipoic acid, n-acetylcysteine, coenzyme Q10, L-carnitine, and all B vitamins, plus the minerals selenium, zinc, and chromium. No iron, copper, or manganese would be added to this supplement. The reasons for not adding iron, copper, or manganese are that these trace minerals, when combined with vitamin C, produce excessive amounts of free radicals. In addition, in the presence of antioxidants these minerals are absorbed from the small intestine in greater amounts and can increase the body's store of free iron, copper, or manganese. Increased free iron and copper stores in the body have been linked to several chronic diseases, including cancer. We recommend that radiation workers and pilots and attendants of civilian and military aircrafts take four capsules per day, two in the morning and two in the evening with meals, throughout their lifetime in order to reduce the potential risk of radiation damage, including cancer.

A well-designed clinical study of micronutrient preparations and the reduction of cancer risk in radiation and aircraft workers would involve the participation of a multicenter trial at the cost of millions of dollars over ten to twenty years. At this time it is not possible to conduct such a study in patients receiving diagnostic radiation procedures or in radiation workers. Until such a study is completed the proposed micronutrient preparations for tissue protection appears to be one of the most rational choices to reduce the adverse effects of low doses of radiation. Adopt these recommendations only after consultation with a physician.

CONCLUDING REMARKS

The growing use of X-ray-based equipment in the diagnosis of human diseases has raised concerns about the potential of such procedures in increasing the risk of cancer and somatic and heritable mutations. These risks also exist in radiation workers, the number of which have increased proportionally with the increased use of diagnostic radiation procedures. The initial physical concept of radiation protection involved lead shielding, increased distance between the radiation source and radiation workers or patients, and reduction of radiation-exposure time. In addition, the concept of ALARA (as low as reasonably achievable) continues to be supported for reducing the doses from diagnostic radiation procedures in patients, and suggestions are being made to reduce overuse of diagnostic radiation procedures.

At present there is no tissue-radiation protection strategy available for patients receiving diagnostic doses, radiation workers, frequent flyers, and pilots and crew of civilian and military aircraft. Because radiation exposure generates excessive amounts of free radicals, and since antioxidants neutralize free radicals, the use of the proposed micronutrient preparation may be one of the best methods of providing tissue-radiation protection against low doses of radiation. This implementation would help to extend the concept of ALARA to PAMARA (protection as much as reasonably achievable). The proposed micronutrient preparation has not yet been tested by a randomized, double-blind, placebo-controlled clinical trial, but it still appears to be one of the most rational choices for reducing the potential damage caused by diagnostic doses of radiation. Adopt these recommendations only after consultation with a physician.

6 Why Do Controversies Exist about Antioxidants in Cancer Prevention?

Micronutrients that have been used in cancer-prevention and -treatment studies include antioxidants, B vitamins, vitamin D, and the mineral selenium. Despite extensive laboratory and human studies on cancer prevention and treatment with micronutrients, the incidence of this disease has not significantly changed and, in fact, appears to have risen. For example, a decade ago the annual incidence of cancer was about 1.2 million new cases per year; in 2009 it was estimated by the American Cancer Society to be about 1.5 million new cases per year.

As mentioned previously, the U.S. mortality rate from cancer has not changed significantly since 1950, despite the development of new chemotherapeutic agents and radiation therapy. In order to reduce the incidence of cancer, supplementation with multiple micronutrients, together with changes in diet and lifestyle, is essential. Although there is a uniform opinion among the scientific and medical communities about the value of modifications in diet and lifestyle for reducing the incidence of cancer, there is no such agreement about the value of micronutrients, including antioxidant supplements. Conflicting reports on the effects of micronutrients have often been reported in newspapers, magazines, and Internet-based media. For example, one day you might read that vitamin E reduces the risk of cancer, and another day you will read that vitamin E may increase the risk of some cancers. Many medical professionals are confused by these contradictory observations and consequently do not feel comfortable recommending them to their patients. We now look at the bases for these contradictions, as well as how they might be resolved.

1. **Reliance on the results of laboratory studies.** Laboratory studies on cancer prevention are generally performed on animals as well as on tissue-culture (cells grown in petri dishes) models, using only one micronutrient. These studies have consistently shown the beneficial effects of a micronutrient in cancer prevention, but only a potential benefit in humans. Human cancer results from the complex interaction between dietary, lifestyle, and environmental agents. In addition, the internal oxidative environment is elevated in high-risk populations (such as tobacco smokers) that are often used in cancer-prevention studies. The use of a single micronutrient in cancer-prevention studies in humans has produced inconsistent results. Therefore, in our opinion, relying only on the laboratory data from animal and tissue-culture studies for recommending or not recommending micronutrients for cancer prevention in humans has little scientific rationale.

2. **Reliance on the findings of epidemiologic studies.** Epidemiologic, or survey-type, studies are important for establishing an association between a diet rich in antioxidants and reduced risk of cancer. These studies are highly complex and have inherent difficulties in accounting for all the variations in diet, lifestyle, and environment that have an impact on cancer incidence. Therefore, in our opinion, the results of epidemiologic studies alone should not be used for recommending or not recommending micronutrients for cancer prevention.

3. **Reliance on the findings of clinical studies in which only one micronutrient is used.** Most clinical studies have utilized only one antioxidant to determine if there is a reduced risk of

cancer in high-risk populations, such as heavy tobacco smokers. These studies have often revealed an increased risk of cancer in the antioxidant-treated group compared with those who received a placebo (no antioxidant treatment). The internal oxidative environment is high among the populations at high risk for developing cancer. Individual antioxidants can be oxidized in such an environment to become pro-oxidants that can increase the risk of cancer. The use of a preparation of multiple micronutrients might prohibit this reaction. Therefore, in our opinion, the results of these studies based on a single antioxidant should not be used for recommending or not recommending multiple micronutrients for cancer prevention.

4. **Failure to distinguish between the effects of preventive and therapeutic doses of antioxidants.** In the interpretations of all clinical and laboratory studies, the distinction between the effects of preventive doses (which have no effect on the growth of cancer or normal cells) and therapeutic doses (which inhibit the growth of cancer cells but not of normal cells) has not been made. This distinction is important, because preventive doses of antioxidants may protect cancer cells against damage produced by radiation therapy and/or chemotherapy, whereas therapeutic doses of antioxidants may increase the effectiveness of other therapeutic agents on cancer cells.

5. **Reliance on publication of meta-analysis (re-analysis) of already published studies.** In recent years meta-analysis publications have become very popular. The re-analysis of published results on the role of micronutrients in cancer prevention is very important. However, it must be done critically and examine the results of only those studies that are similar in design, antioxidant type, form, and dose. Unfortunately, most re-analysis studies have summarized previous studies that were flawed to begin with, and, as expected, came to the same conclusions. Relying on conclusions obtained from this form of re-analysis of old data is inaccurate.

MICRONUTRIENT CONTROVERSIES
IN HUMAN CANCER PREVENTION

In order to understand the controversies surrounding the value of micronutrients in human cancer prevention, it is essential to discuss the relevance of the results of laboratory, epidemiologic, and intervention studies in human cancer prevention.

Laboratory Studies Using
Micronutrients in Cancer Prevention

Before performing cancer-prevention studies with micronutrients in humans, it was essential to conduct experiments in the laboratory using animals (primarily rats and mice) and tissue culture (normal and cancer cells growing in petri dishes). In laboratory studies animals or cells are treated with one micronutrient, generally an antioxidant, prior to administration of a cancer-causing substance. At the end of the study period the incidence of cancer is determined. Numerous laboratory studies have confirmed that a single antioxidant reduces the risk of chemical- and radiation-induced cancer. A few examples of these studies are described here.

Cancer-Prevention Studies on
Normal Cells in Cell Culture

Tissue-culture systems (normal or cancer cells growing in petri dishes) provide a unique opportunity to evaluate the anti-cancer properties of antioxidants in a cost- and time-effective manner. In addition, detailed studies on how antioxidants act at the cellular and genetic levels can only be performed effectively in tissue culture because such studies could not be carried out in animal models due to the inherent complexity of the whole organism. In 1982, Dr. K. N. Prasad, while working at the University of Colorado Medical Center in Denver, identified alpha-tocopheryl succinate (vitamin E succinate) as the most effective form of vitamin E in reducing the growth of cancer cells and causing cancer cell death; other forms of vitamin E were found to be ineffective (Prasad et al. 2003; Prasad and Edwards-Prasad 1982). Scientists have reported that vitamin E succinate reduced the incidence of chemical- and ion-izing radiation–induced cancer in cells growing in petri dishes (Borek et al. 1986; Radner and Kennedy 1986). Beta-carotene also reduced the incidence of chemical- and ionizing radiation–induced cancer in cell culture. Natural beta-carotene has been found to be more effective than synthetic beta-carotene in reducing the incidence of radiation-induced cancer (Kennedy and Krinsky 1994). N-acetylcysteine (NAC), a glutathione-elevating agent, markedly inhibited estrogen-induced can-cer in cell culture (Venugopal et al. 2008). From this and other cell-culture studies, it is very clear that antioxidants have the potential to reduce the incidence of cancer in humans.

The mechanisms of cancer prevention by antioxidants may involve neutralization of free radicals and changes in genetic activity. The results of cell-culture studies cannot readily be extrapolated to animals or humans with respect to antioxidant type, dose, or dose schedule. Before performing human studies, it was essential to demonstrate that antioxidants can prevent cancer formation in animals. Some of these are described here.

Cancer-Prevention Studies on Animals

The role of antioxidants in cancer prevention was demonstrated in ani-mals long before any human study. A two-stage model of cancer forma-tion was developed and utilized to investigate how normal cells become cancer cells and to determine the efficacy of antioxidants in cancer prevention (Boutwell 1983). The overwhelming majority of studies performed using this model suggested that supplementation with high doses of individual antioxidants, such as vitamin C, vitamin E, reti-noids, and carotenoids, reduced the risk of chemical-induced tumors (Cohen and Bhagavan 1995; Prasad and Edwards-Prasad 1992; Hill and Grubbs 1982; Krinsky 1989; Santamaria, Bianchi, and Mobilio 1988). Among the various forms of vitamin E, vitamin E succinate was the most effective in reducing the growth of cancer cells (Prasad et al. 2003; Prasad and Edwards-Prasad 1982). In the animal model the com-bination of vitamin E, selenium, and lycopene was found to be effective in reducing the risk of prostate cancer, whereas the combination of vitamin E and selenium was ineffective (Venkateswaran 2009). The results of this study suggest that the addition of other antioxidants may be necessary to reduce the risk of cancer in general and prostate cancer in particular. In pregnant mice who lacked the p53 tumor-suppressor gene (called p53-knockout mice), prenatal supplementation with vitamin E inhibited the risk of cancer in the offspring by reducing the free radical–induced damage to DNA (Chen, Squire, and Wells 2009). The result of the combined effect of vitamin E and selenium is consistent with the results of the Selenium and Vitamin E Cancer Prevention Trial (SELECT) in which the combination of vitamin E and selenium was found to be ineffective in reducing the risk of prostate cancer (Lippman et al. 2009). The data from the above animal studies also suggested that the addition of other antioxidants may be necessary to reduce the risk of cancer in general and prostate cancer in particular.

According to one study, dihydrolipoic acid, a reduced form of alpha-lipoic aid, significantly reduces the incidence chemical-induced cancer (Wang, Yang, and Pan 2008; Ho et al. 2007). In genetic models of mice with breast- and intestinal-cancer-causing genes inserted, supplementation with alpha-lipoic acid did not affect the incidence of breast or colon cancer (Rossi et al. 2008). The reasons for these contradictory results between genetic model of cancer and chemical-induced cancer in animals remain unknown. It is possible that the susceptibility of the animals with inserted oncogenes may not be related to increased oxidative stress in the formation of cancer. It is equally possible that other antioxidants rather than alpha-lipoic acid alone may be needed to reduce the incidence of cancer in these genetic models.

The effect of n-acetylcysteine (NAC) on cancer prevention in animals has produced inconsistent results. For example, in a mouse genetic model for lymphoma, supplementation with NAC inhibited the incidence and the size of chemical-induced tumors (Reliene and Schiestl 2006); however, it did not change the incidence of chemical-induced liver tumors (Balansky et al. 2002). In the genetic models of skin tumors, supplementation with NAC did not affect the incidence of cancer but reduced the size of tumors (Martin et al. 2001). Supplementation with NAC also did not affect the incidence of chemical-induced breast cancer (Lubet et al. 1997), but it did inhibit the incidence of chemical-induced (by urethane) lung cancer (De Flora, Rossi, and De Flora 1986). These results suggest that the cancer-preventive effect of NAC treatment alone is inconsistent. On the other hand, vitamin E in combination with NAC was more effective in reducing the incidence of chemical-induced cancer than the individual agents (Hao et al. 2009). Thus, the effects of NAC in reducing chemical- or genetic-induced cancers in rodent models are variable depending on the type of tumor and tumor-inducing agents. It is interesting to note that both NAC and alpha-lipoic acid, when used individually, produced inconsistent results even in animal models. Supplementation with coenzyme Q10 has shown reduced chemical-induced (by azoxymethane) precancerous changes in the colon of male rats (Sakano et al. 2006).

A few studies found that certain antioxidants at very high doses when used individually may increase the risk of cancer. For example, vitamin E at very high doses (40 g per person per day) increased the risk of chemical-induced cancer in the small intestine of mice (Toth and Patil 1983). Vitamin C, in the form of sodium ascorbate, enhanced the risk of chemical-induced bladder cancer in rats when given in a high dose (Fukushima et al. 1988); the increased osmolarity of urine caused chronic irritation in the bladder, which may account for the increased risk of cancer. The use of such high doses of antioxidants in cancer prevention should be avoided.

Most published studies using animals have relied on a single dietary or endogenous antioxidant and have yielded sometimes inconsistent results. The efficacy of a mixture of dietary and endogenous antioxidants in reducing the incidence of chemical-induced cancer in animals has never been tested. From animal studies, we can conclude that a mixture of antioxidants has the potential to reduce the risk of cancer in humans.

Although animals are useful for determining the efficacy of antioxidants in cancer prevention, the results obtained from these studies cannot be extrapolated to humans because the absorption, tissue distribution, biological turnover, and metabolism of these antioxidants in animals are totally different from those in humans. For example, unlike humans, most mammals (except guinea pigs) make their own vitamin C, which could have an impact on the dose and efficacy of antioxidants. Laboratory animal diets do not vary much day to day, but the human diet can vary markedly from one day to another in the same individual, and from one person to another.

The fact that naturally occurring nontoxic agents, such as dietary and endogenous antioxidants, can reduce the risk of cancer induced by cancer-causing substances (tumor initiators with or without tumor promoters) created a lot of excitement among nutritionists and cancer researchers. The search for similar effects of antioxidants in cancer prevention in humans began.

Human Cancer-Prevention Studies with Micronutrients

Cancer-prevention studies using micronutrients in humans can be performed by two distinct methods: epidemiology (survey-type study) and intervention (clinical study in which a preventive agent is administered daily for the entire period). There are two experimental designs for epidemiologic studies: retrospective case-control study and prospective case-control study.

Retrospective case-control study: The design of this study involves the analysis of the past history of dietary intake in cancer patients compared with that in age- and gender-matched healthy people. From this comparison the association between dietary factors and the incidence of cancer is estimated. The data on the history of dietary intake is obtained from the participants through questionnaires. From these data the amounts of micronutrients (such as vitamins A, C, D, and E; beta-carotene; and selenium) and the levels of fat and fiber are determined using appropriate nutrition-related computer software. Using these epidemiologic experimental designs, several studies (Prasad, Cole, and Hovland 1998; Hennekens 1994; Buring and Hennekens 1995) concluded that diets rich in antioxidants but low in fat and high in fiber were associated with reduced risk of cancer.

Prospective case-control study: The design of this study involves an analysis of dietary intake from diet records in which participants write down every meal content and amount every day for the entire study period (which could last for a few years). From the dietary records the amounts of micronutrients (such as vitamins A, C, D, and E; beta-carotene; and selenium) and the levels of fat and fiber are determined using appropriate nutrition-related computer software. The data on dietary records are more reliable than those on dietary history; however, it is difficult to estimate the true amount of fruits, vegetables, fats, and fiber present in each meal, and these estimated amounts are used to determine the levels of micronutrient intake among participants. Therefore, the value of micronutrients obtained from this method cannot be considered reliable. Other inherent problems are similar to those described for retrospective case-control studies. The results of these studies alone should not be used to formulate any recommendation to the public.

EXAMPLES OF EPIDEMIOLOGIC STUDIES ON ANTIOXIDANTS AND CANCER PREVENTION

Epidemiologic studies have suggested that consumption of fruits and vegetables and foods rich in carotene and lycopene may reduce the risk of ovarian cancer (Koushik et al. 2005). A diet low in fat and high in fiber from fruits and vegetables and regular modest consumption of alcohol is associated with reduced risk of benign prostatic hyperplasia (BPH) (Kristal et al. 2008). Studies have also estimated that eating fruits and vegetables can reduce the risk of cancer by about 30 percent (Rodrigues, Bouyon, and Alexandre 2009). Another epidemiologic study showed that eating one or more apples a day was associated with a reduced risk of colorectal cancer. This effect was not observed with other fruits (Jedrychowski and Maugeri 2009). In a prospective study involving 295

cases of breast cancer and 295 control menopausal women, the plasma
levels of retinol, retinyl palmitate, alpha-carotene, beta-carotene, beta-
cryptoxanthin, lutein, lycopene, total carotenoids, alpha-tocopherol,
and gamma-tocopherol were measured. The results showed that beta-
carotene, lycopene, and total carotene were lower in cases compared to
controls. The risk of developing breast cancer was inversely proportional
to the level of beta-carotene in plasma (Sato et al. 2002). However, in
another study the incidence of breast cancer among women was lower
if they had higher blood levels of alpha-carotene but not other carotenoids (Tamimi et al. 2005; Kabat et al. 2009). In a review of six clinical trials and twenty-five epidemiologic studies researchers concluded
that beta-carotene supplementation was not associated with decreased
risk of lung cancer (Gallicchio et al. 2008). On the contrary, in the
VITamines And Lifestyle (VITAL) cohort study researchers observed
that long-term intake of beta-carotene, retinol, or lutein was associated
with an increased risk of lung cancer (Satia et al. 2009). In Brazilian
women dietary intake of folate, vitamin B_6, or vitamin B_{12} had no overall association with breast-cancer risk; however, dietary intake of high
levels of folate was associated with an increased risk of breast cancer in
premenopausal women (Ma et al. 2009).

Increased intake of dietary flavonoids was associated with reduced
risk of lung cancer; however, another study reported no association
between individual or multiple-flavonoid intake and the risk of breast,
ovarian, colorectal, lung, and endometrial cancer (Wang et al. 2009). A
recent study has reported that intake of lycopene, and lycopene through
diet, is associated with decreased risk of prostate cancer (Ellinger et
al. 2009). In the Women's Health Initiative (WHI) involving 133,614
postmenopausal women, the dietary intake of antioxidants, carotenoids,
and vitamin A were not associated with a reduction in ovarian-cancer
risk (Thomson et al. 2008). During eight years of follow-up involving
56,007 French women, the breast-cancer risk in those who ingested
high levels of alpha-linolenic acid (ALA, a form of fatty acid) derived
from fruits, vegetables, and vegetable oil had a lower risk of breast
cancer than those who did not consume ALA (Thiebaut et al. 2009).

However, if ALA from nut mixes and processed foods was consumed, the risk of breast cancer was greater. This suggests that other protective substances in the fruits and vegetables, such as antioxidants, may be necessary to observe the protective effect of ALA. In addition, the risk of breast cancer was lower among women who had the highest level omega-3 fatty acids. Thus, epidemiologic studies examining dietary intake of antioxidants, fat, and fiber or B vitamins alone have produced conflicting results. This may be due to the fact that each of these nutrient groups contributes to reduction in cancer incidence to differing degrees; therefore, consistent results cannot be obtained by separate analysis. In addition, human diets contain agents that can produce opposite effects on cancer risk. For example, antioxidants and fiber are considered cancer-protective substances in the diet, whereas diets rich in fat, meat, calories, and nitrites may increase the risk of cancer. Dietary antioxidants can also influence the metabolism of ingested or inhaled mutagens and carcinogens (Anderson et al. 1985; Conney et al. 1991). These reasons may be why the results of studies on diets that are rich in fruits and vegetables, containing high levels of antioxidants, and are low in fat and high in fiber consistently showed cancer-protective effects.

There are several problems inherent in the above method of studying the role of micronutrients in cancer prevention in humans. For example, it is difficult to recall with any degree of accuracy what kind of diet and how many fruits and vegetables participants consumed during the past week, not to mention the past month or year. In addition, dietary habits (such as consumption of fruits, vegetables, fat, and fiber) and lifestyle (such as smoking) that can affect cancer incidence vary widely from one individual to another. These variables are impossible to control during the study period. Therefore, the positive or negative results obtained from survey-type study cannot be considered reliable for determining the value of micronutrients in cancer prevention. The survey-type study is a powerful method for raising questions about the association between micronutrients and cancer risk, but the results alone should not be used to formulate any recommendation to the public.

Despite the problems associated with epidemiologic studies, these studies continue to be used to investigate the relationship between micronutrients and cancer risk. The contradictory results about the value of micronutrients continue to be published and propagated by media outlets, giving the impression of a cause-and-effect relationship between a micronutrient and cancer risk. We question the overuse of the survey-type study in analyzing the relationship between micronutrients and cancer incidence, and caution that we should not rely on their results until they are confirmed by clinical trials.

Interventional (Clinical) Trials

Interventional trials are the best way of establishing a relationship between micronutrients and cancer prevention beyond any reasonable doubt. However, several points must be considered while designing clinical trials in order to obtain meaningful results. These are:

1. Selection of individuals who are at high risk for developing cancer
2. Levels of the body's oxidative environment in high-risk individuals
3. Selection of micronutrients (single versus multiple), their doses, and dose schedule
4. Sample size and total period of study
5. Study end points
6. Randomized, double-blind, placebo-control design

Selection of individuals who are at high risk. Unlike in animal studies, we do not use a cancer-causing agent to induce cancer in humans. Therefore, researchers use humans who are at high risk for developing cancer for investigating the efficacy of a potential cancer-preventive agent. Examples of such individuals are heavy tobacco smokers, cancer survivors (who have an elevated risk of recurrence of primary tumors, and the development of new cancer that is induced by the treatment agents), and individuals who have a family history of cancer (such as women with mutated BRCA1 and BRCA2 breast-cancer genes).

Levels of the body's oxidative environment in high-risk individuals. Suppose individuals who are heavy tobacco smokers are selected for a cancer-prevention study. Tobacco smoke generates excessive amounts of free radicals in the body and depletes antioxidants from the body, creating a high oxidative environment (Kiyosawa et al. 1990; Reznick et al. 1992; Duthie, Arthur, and James 1991; Schectman, Byrd, and Hoffmann 1991). Cancer survivors also have a high oxidative environment, because most cancer-treatment agents are known to increase oxidative stress in the body.

Selection of micronutrients (single versus multiple), their doses, and dose schedule. Knowing that the bodies of the tobacco smokers have a high oxidative environment, selection of a single antioxidant for a cancer-prevention study would be undesirable because this antioxidant, once it enters the bloodstream, would be damaged by free radicals. Damaged antioxidants act as free radicals (pro-oxidant) rather than as antioxidants. This then could increase the risk of cancer. The same effect will not happen if the antioxidant is part of a multiple-antioxidant preparation, because the antioxidant will be protected from free-radical damage by other antioxidants. The use of a single antioxidant is not appropriate for another reason: laboratory experiments have shown that low doses of antioxidants may stimulate the growth of some cancer cells (Prasad and Kumar 1996). For instance, it is possible that some heavy tobacco smokers may already have undetectable lung cancer. In this case administration of a single antioxidant at low doses may increase the proliferation of the residual cancer cells. However, if the same dose of antioxidant is present in a multiple-antioxidant preparation, the growth of cancer cells might be inhibited. This is because antioxidants act synergistically in a multiple-antioxidant preparation.

The references for this section have been provided in a review (Prasad, Cole, and Prasad 2002).

Different types of free radicals are produced in the body. The body also has multiple dietary and endogenous antioxidants to destroy these free radicals when produced in excessive amounts. Each antioxidant has a different affinity for each of these free radicals, depending on the cellular environment. The gradient of oxygen pressure varies within cells and tissues. Vitamin E is more effective in neutralizing free radicals in reduced oxygen pressure, whereas beta-carotene and vitamin A are more effective in higher oxygen pressure. Vitamin C is necessary to protect cellular components immersed in water against free-radical damage, whereas carotenoids and vitamins A and E protect cellular components in lipid environments. Vitamin C also plays an important role in maintaining cellular levels of vitamin E by recycling damaged (oxidized) vitamin E to the antioxidant (reduced) form. Also, the DNA damage produced by oxidized vitamin C can be prevented by vitamin E. The form and type of vitamin E used are also important to improve its beneficial effects. Various organs of rats are known to selectively absorb the natural form of vitamin E; therefore, this form is recommended in multiple-vitamin preparations. It has been established that alpha-tocopheryl succinate (alpha-TS) is the most effective form of vitamin E; therefore this form of vitamin E is recommended in multiple-vitamin preparations. The natural forms of vitamin E and beta-carotene are more effective than their synthetic counterparts. For example, natural beta-carotene reduced radiation-induced transformation in mammalian cells in culture, but synthetic beta-carotene did not. Antioxidants are distributed differently in various organs and even within the same cells. Selenium, a cofactor of glutathione peroxidase, acts as an antioxidant. Therefore, selenium supplementation together with other dietary and endogenous antioxidants is also important.

Glutathione, an endogenously made antioxidant, represents a potent protective agent against oxidative damage in the cells. It catabolizes H_2O_2 and anions and is very effective in neutralizing peroxynitrite, a powerful form of free radical derived from nitrogen. Therefore, increasing the intracellular levels of glutathione is essential for the protection of various components within the cells. Oral supplementation with glutathione does not significantly increase its levels in the plasma of humans, suggesting that this antioxidant is completely destroyed in the gastrointestinal tract. N-acetylcysteine is not destroyed in the intestinal tract, and when it enters the cells, n-acetyl is removed and cysteine is used to make glutathione. Alpha-lipoic acid, an endogenously made antioxidant, also increases the level of glutathione in the cells. Therefore, in order to optimally increase the level of glutathione, it is necessary to use both n-acetylcysteine and alpha-lipoic acid in a multiple-vitamin preparation. Coenzyme Q10, an endogenously made antioxidant, is needed by the mitochondria to generate energy. In addition, it scavenges peroxy radicals faster than alpha-tocopherol, and, like vitamin C, can regenerate vitamin E. Therefore, the addition of coenzyme Q10 in a multiple-vitamin preparation is essential for optimal benefit. These studies suggest that the use of one or two antioxidants to investigate the role of antioxidants in reducing cancer incidence has no scientific rationale. Therefore, for any human cancer-prevention study, we propose the utilization of a multiple-micronutrient preparation containing dietary and endogenous antioxidants, all B vitamins, vitamin D, and appropriate minerals.

The doses of all ingredients in a multiple-vitamin preparation, especially dietary and endogenous antioxidants, can be higher than RDA values but must be nontoxic.

Most clinical studies have utilized a once-a-day dose schedule. Taking micronutrients once a day creates significant fluctuations in their levels in the body. This is because the biological half-lives (time needed to remove 50 percent from the body) of micronutrients vary markedly, depending on their lipid or water solubility. A twofold difference in the levels of vitamin E succinate can produce marked alterations in the expression profiles of several genes in neuroblastoma cells in culture (Prasad, unpublished observation). Therefore, taking micronutrients once a day can create genetic stress in the cells that may compromise the efficacy of the micronutrient supplementation after long-term consumption. Therefore, we recommend taking the supplements twice a day in order to maintain a more consistent level of antioxidants in the body.

Sample size and total period of study. The latent period, even in high-risk populations, may be long; therefore, a study period of at least five to seven years should be selected in order observe any significant difference in cancer incidence. The sample size must be large in order to detect sufficient numbers of individuals with cancer, to provide a meaningful conclusion.

Study end points. In studies with lung cancers the primary end point is cancer. The secondary end point could be quality of life.

Randomized, double-blind, placebo-control design. In this type of study, the individuals are randomly divided into two groups: one receives daily oral dosing of a multiple-micronutrient supplement, and the other receives a placebo (pills with no nutrient) for the entire period of study. At the end of the study period the number of individuals with cancer in the micronutrient-treated group is compared with the number in the placebo group.

Examples of Interventional Trials

The results of several clinical studies on micronutrients in cancer prevention among high-risk populations have been published in prestigious scientific journals. Unfortunately, none of these studies have considered the main issues discussed above; therefore, the results have been inconsistent. Some examples of these clinical trials are described here, because they are often quoted to support the case for not recommending antioxidants in cancer prevention.

Use of one or two dietary antioxidants. In some clinical studies, oral administration of synthetic beta-carotene once a day at a dose of 20 mg per day increased the incidence of lung cancer, prostate cancer, and stomach cancer among male heavy tobacco smokers (Albanes et al. 1995; Omenn et al. 1996; The Alpha-tocopherol Beta-carotene Cancer Prevention Study Group 1994). This increase in cancer incidence could have been predicted, because beta-carotene in the high oxidative environment of a heavy smoker's body would be damaged by free radicals and would then act as a free radical (pro-oxidant) rather than as an antioxidant. In contrast, the same dose of beta-carotene does not have a significant effect on cancer incidence in normal populations who have a lower internal oxidative environment (Hennekens et al. 1986).

Consumption of vitamin E increased the incidence of secondary (new) cancer after cancer therapy in cancer survivors (Bairati et al. 2005), because the oxidative environment is also high in the bodies of cancer survivors. The causal relationship between vitamin E supplementation and increased mortality (Miller et al. 2005) has been contradicted by another statistical analysis study (Gerss and Kopcke 2009). In another study daily supplementation with vitamin C (4,000 mg) and vitamin E (400 mg) also failed to reduce the risk of colon polyps, but when they were combined with a high-fiber diet (more than 12 g per day), there was a significant reduction in the incidence of recurrence of polyps (DeCosse, Miller, and Lesser, 1989).

In a randomized, placebo-controlled trial referred to as the Selenium and Vitamin E Cancer Prevention Trial (SELECT), involving 35,553 healthy men from 427 participating sites in the United States, Canada, and Puerto Rico, with a follow-up period of a minimum of seven years and a maximum of twelve years, it was observed that selenium (200 mcg per day) and vitamin E (400 IU per day), alone or in combination, did not reduce the risk of prostate cancer (Lippman et al. 2009).

In a clinical study involving 2,592 cancer survivors (60 percent with head and neck cancer and 40 percent with lung cancer), a two-year supplementation with vitamin A (retinyl palmitate, 300,000 IU daily for one year, and 150,000 IU for the second year) and NAC (600 mg daily for two years), alone or in combination, produces no benefit on the incidence of secondary new tumors (van Zandwijk 2000). This suggests that one or two antioxidants are not sufficient to reduce the risk of cancer. It should be noted that this study utilized unusually high doses of vitamin A that could be toxic after a long-term consumption. Even the dose of NAC in this study was high.

In another study beta-carotene supplementation in patients with low dietary intake of the same antioxidant reduced prostate cancer (Kirsh et al. 2006). High doses of beta-carotene also caused regression of leukoplakia (potentially precancerous lesion in the mouth) (Benner et al. 1993; Garewal 1995).

One study showed that supplementation with vitamin E (50 mg per day) reduces prostate cancer and colorectal cancer, but it increases the incidence of stomach cancer (Albanes et al. 1995). Supplementation with vitamin E (400 IU) produced no effect on prostate-specific antigen (PSA) levels (Hernandez et al. 2005), a marker of prostate cancer; however, high serum levels of vitamin E were associated with reduced prostate cancer incidence (Alkhenizan and Hafez 2007; Weinstein et al. 2007; Weinstein et al. 2005). In another study supplementation with vitamin E at 400 IU a day was associated with a reduced risk of prostate cancer in tobacco smokers, whereas beta-carotene supplementation was associated with reduced risk of this cancer only in smokers who had low levels of beta-carotene (Kirsh et al. 2006).

In a recent clinical study involving 7,627 cancer-free women, vitamin C (500 mg of ascorbic acid daily), a natural source of vitamin E (600 IU of alpha-tocopherol every other day) and beta-carotene (50 mg every other day) supplementation had no impact on cancer incidence or cancer mortality during a follow-up period of 9.4 years (Lin et al. 2009). Using the population of the Alpha-tocopherol, Beta-carotene Cancer Prevention (ATBC) Study of Finnish male smokers, higher blood levels of alpha-tocopherol concentrations were associated with reduced risk of pancreatic cancer (Stolzenberg-Solomon 2009).

Another study showed that supplementation with vitamin A at a dose of 300,000 IU per day for twelve months produced an 11 percent reduction in recurrence of primary non-small-cell lung carcinoma (Pastorino et al. 1993), but this high dose cannot be given for a prolonged period of time because of toxicity. Retinoids also caused regression of oral leukoplakia (a potentially precancerous lesion) and other cancers (Meyskens 1995).

The results of supplementation with one or two antioxidants should not be extrapolated to the effect of the same antioxidants when present in multiple-antioxidant preparations. Nevertheless, many scientists, researchers, physicians, and some publications are promoting the idea that supplementation with antioxidants can be deleterious to your health and should not be taken for cancer prevention.

Use of multiple dietary antioxidants. The administration of the dietary antioxidants vitamin A (40,000 IU), vitamin C (2,000 mg), vitamin E (400 IU), zinc (90 mg), and vitamin B6 (100 mg) per day, in combination with BCG (bacille bilie de Calmette-Guérin) vaccine caused a 50 percent reduction in the recurrence of bladder cancer in five years, in comparison to control patients who received multiple vitamins containing RDA levels of nutrients and BCG (Lamm et al. 1994).

In another study supplementation with antioxidants (vitamin A, 30,000 IU; vitamin C, 1,000 mg; vitamin E, 70 mg) per day reduced the recurrence of colon polyps from 36 to 6 percent (Roncucci et al. 1993); however, consumption of synthetic beta-carotene (25 mg), vitamin C (1,000 mg), and vitamin E (400 mg) per day failed to show any beneficial effects on the recurrence of colon polyps (Greenberg et al. 1994). Daily supplementation of vitamin C (400 mg) and DL-alpha-tocopherol (400 mg) also failed to reduce the recurrence of colon polyps (McKeown-Eyssen et al. 1988). In another study daily supplementation with vitamin C (4,000 mg) and vitamin E (400 mg) also failed to reduce the risk of colon polyps, but when they were combined with a high-fiber diet (more than 12 grams per day) there was significant reduction in the recurrence of polyps (DeCosse, Miller, and Lesser 1989). This study indicated the importance of a high-fiber diet in combination with antioxidants in cancer prevention in high-risk populations.

In the Linxian General Population Nutrition Interventional Trial in China, a preparation of multiple dietary antioxidants (beta-carotene, vitamin E, and selenium at doses two to three times that of the U.S. RDA) reduced mortality by 10 percent and cancer incidence by 13 percent (Blot et al. 1993). The beneficial effects of this supplementation on mortality were still evident up to 10 years after the cessation of supplementation and were consistently greater in younger participants (Qiao 2009).

The combination of vitamins A, C, and E; omega-3 fatty acids; and folic acid significantly reduced the recurrence of colon adenoma in patients after polypectomy (Biasco and Paganelli 1999). In a randomized placebo-controlled trial involving 80 untreated patients with prostate cancer, daily supplementation with vitamin E, selenium, vitamin C, and coenzyme Q10 did not affect serum levels of prostate-specific antigen (Hoenjet et al. 2005).

It is interesting to note that none of above studies utilized endogenous antioxidants such as alpha-lipoic acid, N-acetylcysteine, coenzyme Q10, and L-carnitine. Addition of these antioxidants may have produced consistent beneficial effects on cancer incidence in high-risk populations.

From these studies it appears that supplementation with one or more dietary antioxidants alone may not be sufficient to produce beneficial and consistent effects on reducing the risk of cancer. Inclusion of endogenous antioxidants may be necessary in the design of clinical studies to test the efficacy of antioxidants in cancer prevention.

Cancer Risk after Treatment with Vitamin D and Calcium

In recent years the role of vitamin D alone or in combination with calcium has been evaluated often and yielded inconsistent results. Some studies showed that vitamin D at 1,000 IU per day reduced colorectal cancer (Gorham et al. 2005; Gorham et al. 2007). In another study 400 IU of vitamin D and 1,000 mg of calcium per day produced no effect on colorectal cancer (Wactawski-Wende et al. 2006). In a different study, administration of 400 IU of vitamin D and 1,000 mg calcium per day reduced colorectal cancer but in combination with estrogen increased the risk of this cancer (Ding et al. 2008). In view of the fact that estrogen is known to have tumor-promoting effects and vitamin D has no effect on the activity of estrogen, the above increase in cancer incidence is expected. This could have been avoided by the addition of antioxidants that are known to reduce the effect of tumor promoters.

A recent review of several clinical studies concluded that supplementation with elemental calcium may have a modest effect in reducing the risk of colorectal cancer; however, this approach is not recommended for reducing the risk of colorectal cancer in the general population (Weingarten, Zalmanovici, and Yaphe 2008). Supplementation with elemental 1,000 mg of calcium and 400 IU of vitamin D a day did not reduce the risk of breast cancer (Chlebowski et al. 2008). However, in another study dietary intake of calcium was modestly associated with reduced risk of breast cancer in postmenopausal women (McCullough et al. 2005). In the Wheat Bran Fiber Trial higher intake of calcium (1,068 mg versus 690 mg per day) decreased the risk of recurrence of colorectal adenomas by about 45 percent (Martinez et al. 2002). A possible effect of this treatment was also noted in women with the mutation in the breast cancer gene (mutated BRCA gene). Another study reported that calcium and vitamin D supplementation together reduced the recurrence of colorectal adenomas (Grau et al. 2003). For more consistency in study results, vitamin D and calcium should be used with other micronutrients, such as antioxidants and B vitamins.

Cancer Risk after Treatment with Folate and B Vitamins

Diets rich in folate and vitamins B_6 and B_{12} have been associated with reduced risk of breast cancer and colorectal cancer but have had no association with pancreatic cancer (Harnack et al. 2002; Ishihara et al. 2007; Kune and Watson 2006; Lajous et al. 2006; Zhang 2004). However, supplementation with folic acid alone did not reduce the incidence of colorectal adenomas and may increase the risk of colorectal cancer (Cole et al. 2007). In other studies consumption of folate did not reduce the incidence of colorectal cancer (Logan et al. 2008). In a clinical trial involving 137 patients who underwent polypectomy (removal of polyps), supplementation with 5 mg folate daily reduced the recurrence of colon polyps (Jaszewski 2008). Dietary intake of high amounts of folate and vitamin B_{12} have been independently associated with decreased risk of breast cancer, particularly in postmenopausal women, whereas there is no association between intake of vitamin B_6 and breast cancer in young women (Lajous et al. 2006). In a recent survey-type study, people with low serum levels of folate appeared to be at increased risk of cancer (Yang et al. 2009). Folate and B vitamins can be expected to yield inconsistent results; therefore, we propose combining all B vitamins and folate with multiple micronutrients in our proposed cancer-prevention strategy.

Fat and Fiber

Fiber. Average American diets are low in fiber. A review of published data on supplementation with fiber showed no significant effects on recurrence of colon adenomas, although most epidemiological studies have shown an inverse relationship between consumption of a high-fiber diet and cancer incidence. High-fiber diets contain other micronutrients such as multiple antioxidants; thus, the presence of the other micronutrients may contribute to the protective effect of a high-fiber diet on cancer incidence. A few clinical studies on supplementation with high fiber alone have produced inconsistent results. These studies are described below.

Human survey-type studies have revealed that consumption of a high-fiber diet is associated with a reduced risk of cancer. This protection is thought to be because of fiber's ability to bind increased amounts of intestinal cholesterol, bile acids, and the mutagens and carcinogens that are formed during digestion and eliminate them in the feces. This then reduces intestinal absorption and exposure time of the intestinal cells to these potentially carcinogenic substances. Therefore, it was assumed that only cancer of the intestinal tract would be reduced by this mechanism of action. However, the consumption of high fiber reduced the recurrence of breast cancer. Therefore, additional cancer-protective mechanisms may exist. Indeed, it has been reported that high fiber intake can generate very high (millimolar) levels of butyric acid, a four-carbon fatty acid, with the help of endogenous bacteria that are present in the colon. Being a small fatty acid, butyric acid is absorbed rapidly. Several studies have reported that butyrate and its analog (phenyl butyrate) have exhibited strong anticancer properties against a variety of tumors. Thus, high-fiber diets may provide protection not only against colon cancer but also against other tumors, making these diets essential for our proposed cancer-prevention strategy.

Fat. In the Polyp Prevention Trial dietary intervention, including reduced fat and increased consumption of fruits and vegetables and fiber, produced no effect on prostate-specific antigen and on the incidence of prostate cancer in normal men (Shike et al. 2002). Similarly, adopting a diet low in fat (20 percent of total calories) and high in fiber (18 g per 1,000 kcal) and fruits and vegetables (3.5 serving per 1,000 kcal) did not influence the risk of recurrence of colorectal adenomas (Schatzkin 2000). In contrast to the above observation, another study reported that vitamin A from food with or without supplemental vitamin A and alpha-carotene from food may protect against the recurrence of tumors in nonsmokers and nondrinkers (Steck-Scott et al. 2004). The current dietary guidelines (fruits, vegetables, whole-grain, low-fat dairy, and lean meat) are associated with decreased risk of mortality from all causes (Kant et al. 2000). Supplementation with wheat-bran fiber (13.5 grams per day versus 2 grams per day) did not protect against recurrence of colorectal adenomas (Alberts et al. 2000). Testing the effect of a high-fiber diet, as in the above study—in which difference between the control and experimental groups was only 11.5 grams—may not be sufficient to yield any significant reduction in cancer incidence. Such an interventional trial does not appear to have scientific rationale.

In a multi-institutional, randomized, controlled trial involving 3,088 women previously treated for early stage breast cancer, supplementation with a diet high in vegetables, fruits, and fiber and low in fat did not reduce additional breast cancer development or mortality during a 7.3-year follow-up period (Pierce et al. 2007). The lack of additional micronutrients, such as dietary and endogenous antioxidants, B vitamins, and calcium with vitamin D, may have contributed to the failure to detect the protective effects of high fiber and low fat.

The average American diet consists of about 34.1 percent calories from fat. An interventional study called The Women's Health Initiative Dietary Modification Trial, in which postmenopausal women consumed a low-fat (40 percent) or a high-fat (60 percent) diet showed that a low-fat diet did not reduce the risk of colorectal cancer during 8.1 years of follow-up (Beresford et al. 2006). But in our opinion diets in which fat represents 40 percent of the content should not be considered low fat. Further, a difference of only 20 percent fat may not be sufficient to exert any protective effect on cancer incidence. We would consider a diet that contains no more than 25 percent of calories from fat to be low fat. In addition, the protective effect of low fat alone may be minor, and its cancer-protective effects cannot be adequately assessed in any interventional trial.

Heart Outcomes Prevention Evaluation (HOPE) Trial

The analysis of the results of this trial is included because it is often quoted to support the case for not recommending antioxidants for any health reasons. The study was conducted from December 21, 1993, to April 15, 1999. One of the objectives was to evaluate the efficacy of natural vitamin E (400 IU per day) in reducing the risk of heart disease on patients at least fifty-five years of age and with vascular disease or diabetes, many of whom were heavy cigarette smokers. The analysis of data published in five separate publications revealed inconsistent results.

In the analysis published in 2000 the primary end points were major cardiac events (myocardial infarction, or stroke and death due to coronary artery disease), and the secondary end points were unstable angina, heart failure, revascularization, amputation, and complications of diabetes. No significant effect of vitamin E supplementation on primary or secondary end points was observed (Yusuf et al. 2000).

In the analysis published in 2001, in a subset of the study population, the effect of vitamin E on coronary intima-medial thickness (CIMT), as measured by ultrasound, was evaluated. The results showed that vitamin E supplementation had no effect on the progression of atherosclerosis (Lonn et al. 2001).

In the analysis published in 2002, the primary end points were the same as those in 2000, but the secondary end points included an additional criterion: nephropathy (kidney disease). The results showed that vitamin E had no effect on either the primary or the secondary end points (Lonn et al. 2002).

In the analysis published in 2004, the primary end points were the same as those in the analysis of 2000, but the secondary end points included an additional criterion: clinical proteinuria (kidney disease with protein in the urine). The results showed that in people with mild to moderate renal insufficiency, vitamin E had no effect on primary or secondary end points (Mann et al. 2004).

In the analysis published in 2005 the primary and secondary end points were the same as those in the analysis of 2000. The results showed that vitamin E supplementation had no effect on the primary or most secondary end points; however, it increased the risk of two secondary end points—heart failure by about 13 percent and hospitalization for heart failure by about 21 percent (Lonn et al. 2005).

The analysis of a subpopulation of heavy tobacco smokers revealed that smoking increased the risk of morbidity and mortality among high-risk patients despite treatment with standard medications known to reduce cardiovascular disease (Dagenais 2005). This is consistent with another independent study in which daily consumption of 800 IU of vitamin E increased the levels of oxidative stress markers in heavy smokers (Weinberg et al. 2001). These studies suggest that smoking plays a dominant role in increasing morbidity and mortality. If these major cardiac events increased despite treatment with standard medications given to reduce the risk of heart disease, it is not surprising that administration of vitamin E alone had no significant effect on all primary end points and most secondary end points. Individual antioxidants in high-risk populations, such as heavy tobacco smokers and patients with type II diabetes, may be oxidized because of the high oxidative environment in the body, and thereby act as pro-oxidants rather than antioxidants. Again, the HOPE Trial did not consider the above issues, resulting in no beneficial effects or even the harmful effects of vitamin E on some criteria of heart disease.

Publication of Meta-analysis (Re-analysis of Old Data)

In recent years publications featuring an analysis of old studies on micronutrients and cancer prevention have become very popular. On the surface they appear very impressive because they describe the results from hundreds of thousands of people (the sum of individuals who participated in many studies). The conclusions made by this form of re-analysis of old studies are propagated by the media as if they represent new findings. As a matter of fact, in most studies on micronutrients and cancer prevention or treatment, there are differences in the type of high-risk population and in the type, number, form, dose, dose schedule of micronutrients, end points (type of cancer), and period of observation. Unfortunately, all meta-analysis publications have combined the results of such variable studies on micronutrients and cancer prevention (Hennekens et al. 1996; Bairati et al. 2005; Miller et al. 2005), and their conclusions, unsurprisingly, are the same as the original studies. The re-publication of such studies serves no purpose except to create more confusion among the public and most health professionals.

HOW TO RESOLVE THE PRESENT CONTROVERSIES

The inconsistent results obtained by the use of one or a few dietary or endogenous antioxidants, or of fat and fiber alone in high-risk populations, suggests that such experimental designs are not sufficient to determine the efficacy of micronutrients in cancer prevention. The fate of individual antioxidants in a high-oxidative environment also suggests that the use of a single antioxidant may be counterproductive. The distinction between therapeutic and preventive doses of antioxidants must also be made. Therefore, we propose a clinical study in populations at high risk of developing cancer in which all six points described in the section on interventional trials (see page 120) are considered. We suggest that a multiple-micronutrient preparation including dietary and endogenous antioxidants, together with a low-fat and high-fiber diet and changes in lifestyle (see chapter 7 for details), should be included in any clinical trial on cancer prevention. The dose of antioxidants should be higher than RDA values, but not so high as to be toxic.

The preparation of multiple micronutrients should contain dietary antioxidants, such as vitamin A; natural mixed carotenoids (90 percent beta-carotene); two forms of vitamin E (d-alpha-tocopheryl acetate and d-alpha-tocopheryl succinate, also called vitamin E succinate); vitamin C (calcium ascorbate); and endogenous antioxidants such as R-alpha-lipoic acid, N-acetylcysteine, coenzyme Q10, L-carnitine, vitamin D, and all B vitamins; and minerals such as selenium (selenomethionine), zinc, calcium, magnesium, and chromium. Both vitamin A and beta-carotene were added because beta-carotene, in addition to acting as a precursor of vitamin A, performs unique functions that cannot be produced by vitamin A, and vice versa. For example, beta-carotene increases the expression of the connexin gene, which codes for a gap-junction protein that holds two normal cells together, whereas vitamin A does not produce such an effect. Vitamin A produces differentiation (maturation) in normal and cancer cells, but beta-carotene does not. Beta-carotene is more effective at destroying oxygen radicals than most other antioxidants. Thus, the addition of both vitamin A and beta-carotene may enhance the efficacy of a micronutrient preparation in cancer prevention.

The micronutrient preparation contains two forms of vitamin E. Vitamin E succinate is now considered the most effective form of vitamin E. Vitamin E succinate, which is more soluble than alpha-tocopherol or alpha-tocopheryl acetate, enters the cells more easily, where it is converted to alpha-tocopherol and, thus, provides intracellular protection against oxidative damage. It also has its own unique function as vitamin E succinate, altering the expression of many genes in cancer cells. Therefore, in order to increase the efficacy of vitamin E, the addition of both forms of vitamin E is essential. This micronutrient preparation contains no herbs or herbal antioxidants, because certain herbs may adversely interact with prescription and over-the-counter drugs. In addition, herbal antioxidants do not produce unique antioxidant effects that cannot be produced by antioxidants present in the proposed micronutrient preparation.

This formulation does not contain iron, copper, or manganese, because they are known to combine with vitamin C and produce excessive amounts of free radicals that could reduce the optimal effects of the formulation. In addition, these trace minerals, in the presence of antioxidants, are absorbed more efficiently and could increase body stores. The increased body stores of iron or copper have been associated with an increased risk of some chronic human diseases, including cancer. These micronutrient preparations are commercially available as Cellular Security.

In our proposed study design, the placebo group should not have any dietary recommendation or changes in lifestyle. Dietary and lifestyle compliances can be monitored by questionnaires, whereas the compliances for the micronutrient group can be monitored by measuring plasma levels of selected micronutrients every six months. This will test the efficacy of all three components together (micronutrients, diet, and lifestyle). In a different study to determine the efficacy of micronutrient supplements alone, the placebo group would have the same recommendations for changes in diet and lifestyle as those for micronutrient supplement group.

One may argue that this experimentally designed clinical study is complicated because at the end of the study we may not know which particular micronutrient is responsible for cancer reduction. This argument may not be valid, because the primary aim of any clinical study is to achieve success in reducing the risk of cancer. For a mechanistic study on micronutrients, animal and cell-culture models are most suitable.

CONCLUDING REMARKS

Despite nearly two decades of randomized, double-blind, placebo-controlled, and nonrandomized clinical trials primarily conducted with a single dietary antioxidant and in high-risk populations, controversy still exists about the usefulness of antioxidant supplements in reducing the risk of cancer. The results of these clinical trials have varied from no effects to beneficial effects to harmful effects. We have critically examined the results of these studies and concluded that the present trends in clinical research, in which a single antioxidant is used to evaluate the efficacy of antioxidants in reducing the risk and cancer, lack scientific rationale, and, therefore, have not yielded consistent beneficial effects. We have provided potential reasons for the controversies, as well as our rationale for the need for a shift in the design of clinical studies from using one antioxidant alone to using multiple micronutrients, including both dietary and endogenous antioxidants, together with a low-fat and high-fiber diet. The efficacy of the proposed experimental design can be tested in populations at high risk of developing cancer.

7 Proposed Micronutrients and Lifestyle Recommendations

Cancer can occur spontaneously in individuals who have no known risk factors. Those who have a higher risk of developing cancer, such as tobacco smokers, cancer survivors, and those with a family history of cancer, develop tumors earlier and with increased frequency. At present, most doctors, researchers, and health professionals agree that avoiding exposure to environmental carcinogens and making changes in the diet and lifestyle may be useful in reducing the risk of cancer; however, there is disagreement about the value of micronutrients in cancer prevention. In chapter 6 we discussed the reasons for this disagreement and suggested the types of clinical studies that are needed to resolve them. Until such clinical studies are completed, we suggest that most individuals should consider adopting our proposed recommendations after consultation with their doctors or other health care professionals who are knowledgeable about nutrition and cancer. Here are our recommendations, each of which are equally important for reducing the risk of cancer.

1. Avoid exposure to known environmental carcinogens
2. Change dietary habits
3. Change lifestyle
4. Consume a daily multiple-micronutrient preparation containing dietary and endogenous antioxidants

AVOID EXPOSURE TO KNOWN ENVIRONMENTAL CARCINOGENS

The ultraviolet (UV) light from the sun, ionizing radiation from radon gas in certain regions of the country, high levels of ozone in the air, and small amounts of cancer-causing substances in the water supply represent environmental sources of potential carcinogens. Therefore, it is essential that we try to minimize the exposure to these toxic agents. This recommendation has been in existence for a long period of time, but it has had no impact on cancer incidence. It is very difficult to convince people to change their behavior; for example, many people continue to expose themselves to an excessive amount of sun without adequate protection. Furthermore, we often have no control over the levels of cancer-causing substances that are present in the environment. It is also possible the cancer risk from these environmental carcinogens cannot be minimized without the aid of micronutrient supplements and changes in diet and lifestyle.

Sunbathing

Sunbathing and suntanning are very popular. Excessive exposure to sun causes skin cells to make greater amounts of dark pigment, which creates a tan. Although this may achieve a desired cosmetic effect, UV light–tanned skin is at a higher risk for developing skin cancers (basal cell carcinoma, squamous cell carcinoma, and melanoma) several years after exposure. This is because UV light in the sun causes damage to the DNA of the skin cells, making them more vulnerable to accumulating more mutations caused by other agents and eventually leading to cancer. Melanoma is a deadly type of skin cancer, especially if not detected and removed early. There is no effective method of treatment for melanoma once it has spread to other parts of the body, especially the liver and brain. Therefore, it is absolutely essential to avoid exposure to excessive amounts of sunlight without adequate protection (clothing, sunscreen).

CHANGE DIETARY HABITS

Studies on Diet and Cancer Incidence in Different Countries

The United States

The incidence of stomach cancer in the United States has declined because of changing dietary habits and improved food-storage facilities, such as refrigerators. The rates of colon and rectal cancer among Seventh Day Adventists, who are vegetarians, is much lower than among persons who eat meat. In addition, Mormons who do not smoke, drink alcohol, or consume excess caffeine have a lower incidence of colon and rectal cancer. The consumption of a diet low in fiber and high in fat contributes to the increased incidence of various cancers, including breast, colon, and prostate.

Japan

The high incidence of stomach cancer in Japan has been associated with the consumption of spices and pickled food. Japanese people also eat smoked fish, which contains high levels of cancer-causing substances that are present in the smoke. The rate of stomach cancer is markedly lower among Japanese immigrants who adopt Western food habits; however, stomach cancer rates remain high among Japanese immigrants to the United States who continue to follow traditional Japanese dietary habits.

The incidence of breast cancer is low among Japanese women compared with American or European women. This has been attributed to a difference in the fat content of the diet, which also accounts for a difference in the level of circulating blood levels of estrogen. Japanese women, who often eat a low-fat diet, have lower levels of blood estrogen than women in the United States, who usually eat a diet higher in fat. Higher levels of estrogen can act as a tumor promoter and thereby increase the risk of breast cancer.

India

The high rate of oral cancer in India is associated with chewing betel nuts, which contain several cancer-causing agents. The habit of holding dry tobacco leaves and chuna (a substance containing calcium hydroxide) between the lip and gum is associated with an increased incidence of lip cancer. These forms of cancer are not unique to India but are common to all regions where people chew tobacco. The rate of colon cancer among people of Punjab is lower compared with other regions of India, because they eat a diet rich in fiber and low in fat (cellulose, vegetables, fiber, and yogurt).

China

In one province of China there is a high rate of esophageal cancer. This may be related to the low selenium content of the soil. People of this region eat mostly pickled food and only small quantities of fresh fruits and vegetables.

Chile

The high incidence of stomach cancer in Chile appears to be associated with the consumption of food and drinking water that contain relatively high levels of nitrate, a chemical that combines with other chemicals (amines) to form nitrosamine, a potent cancer-causing substance.

Uruguay

In South America, Uruguay has the highest rate of esophageal cancer. The mortality rates from this cancer in males vary from 40 cases per 100,000 in the northeast region to 10 cases per 100,000 in Montevideo, the capital city. Rates in males are about four times higher than in females. Tobacco smoking, alcohol consumption, and drinking maté (a form of tea derived from the herb *Ilex paraguariensis,* which is consumed very hot through a metal straw) in large amounts may contribute to the development of esophageal cancer.

Iceland

The incidence of stomach cancer among Icelanders who consume large quantities of smoked fish and meat is much higher than among those who eat these foods in smaller amounts. Smoked fish contains high levels of hydrocarbons (cancer-causing agents), which are formed during the smoking process.

These studies performed in different countries show that diet plays an important role in determining the risk of cancer. It has been estimated that the dietary factors contribute to about 34 percent of all human cancers. Therefore, a significant portion of the annual incidence of cancer could be reduced by changing our dietary habits.

Recommended Changes in Diet

Most epidemiologic studies support the idea that a low-fat and high-fiber diet rich in fruits and vegetables reduces the risk of cancer. For optimal effect, however, it is essential to include an appropriately prepared multiple-micronutrient preparation containing dietary and endogenous antioxidants, as well as changes in lifestyle.

General dietary recommendations are applicable to all adult individuals irrespective of age, gender, and health risk. They are based on a low-fat and high-fiber diet, and are listed here.

1. Eat three fresh fruits and cooked vegetables daily.
2. Consume about 26 grams of fiber per day from fruits, vegetables, and fiber-rich cereals.
3. Limit fat consumption to 25 percent of total calories (1 gram of fat equals 9 calories). The current average fat consumption in the United States is about 40 percent.
4. Avoid excessive consumption of protein, carbohydrates, and total calories.
5. Restrict foods with high nitrate or nitrite content. Whenever eating such foods, take an antioxidant supplement before the meal (or drink fresh orange juice beforehand).
6. Avoid eating large amounts of charcoal-broiled or smoked meat or fish.
7. Reduce the amount of pickled fruits and vegetables in the diet.
8. Curb consumption of excessive amounts of caffeine-containing beverages (hot or cold).
9. Drink five to six glasses of water every day.

Specific Dietary Recommendation Examples

Breakfast

- Whole-wheat toast or fiber-rich cereals with low-fat or skim milk
- One egg or the white portion of two eggs, cooked
- Fruits rich in carotenoids, such as apricot, mango, peach, grape, or cantaloupe
- Fruits rich in vitamin C, such as oranges, pineapples, strawberries, blueberries, or raspberries
- A cup of coffee (regular or decaffeinated), or black or green tea with or without skim milk

Lunch

- One piece (4 ounces) of skinless chicken or other low-fat meat or fish; vegetarians can substitute with beans and/or soy products
- One whole-wheat roll or toast, or one cup of cooked rice
- Fruits (the same as those suggested for breakfast)
- Two vegetables (select from asparagus, spinach, broccoli, cabbage, green beans, cauliflower, peas, brussels sprouts, corn, and potato)
- Salad containing fruits and vegetables such as spinach, parsley, cucumbers, tomatoes, and grapes, with a small amount of olive oil, low-fat salad dressing of your choice, or lemon juice
- Decaffeinated coffee or tea, or other caffeine-free beverages
- Yogurt with or without fresh fruits for dessert (if desired)

Dinner

The same suggestions as for lunch apply to dinner. In addition, one may enjoy a low-calorie dessert.

Changes in the diet similar to those proposed here have been recommended for decades by the American Cancer Society and other established cancer organizations, but by themselves they have had no impact on the incidence of cancer. It is very difficult to convince people to change their traditional dietary habits in a consistent manner. For optimal effect on cancer-risk reduction, micronutrient supplementation and changes in lifestyle are also essential.

RECOMMENDED
LIFESTYLE CHANGES

Among lifestyle-related factors, tobacco smoking contributes to about one-third of all human cancer. Despite our best educational efforts and laws prohibiting smoking in public places, the number of smokers in the United States has not changed significantly during the past two decades. Additional recommendations for lifestyle changes are listed here.

- Do not smoke. Avoid exposure to secondhand smoke. Do not chew tobacco or tobacco products.
- Avoid exposure to excessive sunlight without adequate protection. Use appropriate sunscreen before going in the sun. Do not use UV light for tanning or hyperbaric therapy (breathing excess of oxygen at high atmospheric pressure) for energy.
- Avoid drinking excessive amounts of alcohol and caffeine-rich beverages.
- Reduce stress through meditation, yoga, or taking regular vacations.
- Exercise three to five days a week for thirty minutes. If you do strenuous aerobic exercise for thirty minutes, take an appropriately prepared micronutrient preparation beforehand.
- Reduce the excessive use of cell phones for a prolonged period of time.

Changes in lifestyle similar to those proposed here have been recommended for decades by the American Cancer Society and other established cancer organizations, but by themselves they have had no impact on the incidence of cancer. It is very difficult to convince people to change their lifestyle in a consistent manner. Micronutrient supplement together with changes in diet and lifestyle are essential for reducing the risk of cancer.

Consume a Daily Multiple-Micronutrient Preparation Containing Dietary and Endogenous Antioxidants

As stated previously, clinical studies in which primarily one micronutrient was used in high-risk populations who had increased risk of developing cancer have produced inconsistent results. In chapter 6 we have made some suggestions for how to resolve this confusion and disagreement. We propose that supplementation with a multiple-micronutrient preparation containing dietary and endogenous antioxidants is necessary for reducing the risk of cancers. We believe these supplements are valuable because:

1. Certain micronutrients, such as antioxidants, vitamin D, and the mineral selenium, perform several biological functions that are pertinent to cancer prevention.
2. Recommendations for changes in diet or lifestyle alone have had no significant impact on reducing the risk of cancer.
3. The increased life span of the U.S. population can increase the risk of age-related cancer.

Certain micronutrients, such as antioxidants, vitamin D, and the mineral selenium, perform several biological functions that are pertinent to cancer prevention: Some of these effects are described here.

Antioxidants as scavengers of free radicals

Excessive production of free radicals may increase the risk of cancer. Both dietary and endogenous antioxidants neutralize free radicals and thereby may reduce the risk of cancer. Multiple antioxidants, rather than a single antioxidant, are needed to destroy all types of free radicals that are produced throughout the body.

Antioxidants prevent the formation of potential cancer-causing substances in the digestive system

Carcinogenic and mutagenic agents are formed during the digestion of food, and antioxidant supplementation can limit the formation of these agents. For example, the consumption of nitrite-rich food (such as bacon, sausage, and cured meat) can form nitrosamines in the stomach at an acid pH through the combination of nitrites and secondary amines already present in the stomach. Nitrosamines are one of the most powerful human carcinogens. The presence of vitamin C or vitamin E in the stomach averts this reaction, which may lower the risk of cancer among those who consume nitrite-rich foods. Diets rich in meat increase the levels of mutagenic substances in the feces compared with vegetarian diets; the presence of high levels of mutagens in the intestinal tract may increase the risk of cancer. Daily intake of vitamin C or vitamin E decreases the amount of mutagenic substances in the feces, and the combination of vitamin C and vitamin E is more effective than either agent alone. Thus, human studies suggest that certain antioxidants can prevent the formation of carcinogens and mutagens in the gastrointestinal tract during digestion.

Antioxidants prevent the conversion of inactive to active carcinogens in the liver

There two forms of carcinogens: direct and indirect. Direct carcinogens, such as X-rays or gamma rays and cancer-causing viruses, can increase the risk of cancer without undergoing any changes in the body. Indirect carcinogens, such as nitrosamine and benzo(a)pyrene, cannot cause cancer until they are converted into their active forms in the liver by oxidation reactions. High levels of antioxidants in the liver may inhibit this reaction and thereby reduce the risk of cancer among those who are absorbing high levels. These inactive carcinogens are then excreted in the urine.

Induction of cell differentiation, growth inhibition, or both in cancer cells

Certain antioxidants at high but nontoxic doses can induce cell differentiation or growth inhibition and cell death, or both, in cancer cells growing in the petri dishes (in vitro studies). The extent of these effects depends on the dose and type of antioxidants and the type of tumor cells. For example, individual retinoids (derivatives of vitamin A) have been found to induce differentiation and growth inhibition in several human and rodent (mice and rats) tumor-cell types. Vitamin E succinate also can produce similar effects in several types of human and rodent tumor cells in culture, but other forms of vitamin E are ineffective. This finding suggests that vitamin E succinate is the most active form of vitamin E in reducing the growth of cancer cells. Beta-carotene and vitamin C also inhibit the growth of some cancer cells in culture. These observations suggest that antioxidants at high doses may convert some newly formed cancer cells to normal-like cells that are not cancerous, and that they can kill cancer cells and reduce their growth.

Antioxidants at low doses can stimulate the growth of cancer cells

In contrast to high doses, low doses of antioxidants can increase the growth of some cancer cells in culture. For example, vitamin C alone at low doses enhances the growth of human leukemia cells and human parotid carcinoma (salivary gland tumor) cells. Beta-carotene alone also can increase the growth of human melanoma cells in cell cultures. The same doses of antioxidants do not encourage the growth of other types of cancer cells. If the same low doses of antioxidants are used in a mixture of antioxidants, they never increase the growth of cancer cells. Thus, the use of a single antioxidant at low doses in cancer prevention trials may be ineffective or even harmful among high-risk populations in which some people may already have pre-cancerous or cancerous cells that are too few to be detected clinically. This prediction of the potentially harmful effect of single antioxidants in high-risk populations was supported in a clinical trial in which beta-carotene alone was used in heavy tobacco smokers.

Antioxidants induce growth inhibition in cancer cells but not in normal cells

As mentioned earlier, vitamin C, vitamin E succinate, beta-carotene, and retinoids at high doses inhibit the growth of cancer cells in humans and rodents. These antioxidants have no growth-inhibiting effects on normal cells, however. This may be due in part to the difference in the uptake of antioxidants between normal and cancer cells. Some tumor cells, such as leukemia, can accumulate higher amounts of these antioxidants than normal cells. The high levels of antioxidants within the tumor cells can lead to cell death, differentiation, or growth inhibition, depending on the concentration of antioxidants, types of antioxidants, and types of cancer cells. In some cases normal and cancer cells may accumulate similar levels of antioxidants; however, tumor cells become more sensitive to antioxidants than normal cells, with respect to cell death or differentiation and growth inhibition.

Effects of interactions between antioxidants on growth of cancer cells

Although extensive studies have been undertaken to investigate the effects of individual antioxidants on the growth and differentiation of tumor cells in culture and in animals, very few studies have been carried out to evaluate the effects of a mixture of several antioxidants on the growth of tumor cells. Our studies show that a mixture of dietary antioxidants (vitamins A, C, and E, and carotenoids) inhibits the growth of cancer cells, although they do not do so when used individually. In general, antioxidants taken together are more effective in suppressing the growth of tumor cells in culture than single antioxidants. In the design of most previous clinical trials among high-risk populations, the importance of synergy between the different antioxidants has been ignored. In our opinion this issue must be considered in the design of any future clinical trials.

Effects of interaction between antioxidants and other physiological substances

Antioxidants not only have a direct effect on tumor cells, individually or in combination, but they also enhance the effects of some physiological agents that are normally made in the body. This could have an important impact on cancer prevention. For example, we have reported that vitamin E succinate and beta-carotene enhance the effect of adenosine 3',5,'-cyclic monophosphate (cAMP), a substance present in all human cells, on the differentiation of the cells of neuroblastoma (a childhood cancer of embryonic nerve cells) in culture. As was discussed earlier, differentiation is the process that converts cancer cells to normal-like cells that are not cancerous. We have also reported that vitamin E succinate also enhances the extent of cAMP-induced differentiation in melanoma cells in culture. Vitamin C, vitamin E succinate, beta-carotene, and retinoids (derivatives of vitamin A) magnify the growth-inhibiting effects of interferon alpha-2b (an immune-stimulant compound that is produced in the body) on human melanoma cells in culture. Retinoids enhance the growth-inhibiting effects of interferon alpha-2a on cervical squamous cell carcinoma in humans. Vitamin E succinate and vitamin C also amplify the growth-inhibiting effects of sodium butyrate (a small fatty acid with anticancer property that is produced in the lower colon with the help of bacteria) on cancer cells.

Antioxidants reduce the action of prostaglandins on cells

High levels of prostaglandins (PGs) act as tumor promoters for some types of cancer. A high-fat diet raises the level of PGs in animals and likewise may increase the incidence of chemical-induced cancer. Anti-inflammatory drugs such as aspirin and indomethacin, which limit the production of PGs, lower the risk of chemical-induced cancer in animals. We have reported that vitamin E succinate inhibits the action of PGE1 in mammalian cells in culture. A combination of vitamin C and vitamin E inhibits production and release of PGE2. In addition, vitamin E in combination with aspirin is more effective at reducing the production of PGs than the individual agents. These results suggest a combination of non-steroidal anti-inflammatory drugs and several antioxidants may lessen the risk of PG-mediated cancer more effectively than individual agents alone.

Antioxidants reduce the incidence
of mutations in normal cells

As we have indicated earlier, all cancers are preceded by mutations (changes in DNA), but not all mutations lead to cancer. Random mutations occur all the time in the body. They are considered risk factors in the development of cancer, and eventually can lead to it. Vitamin C, vitamin E, and beta-carotene prevent mutations caused by X-rays or gamma rays and chemical carcinogens. Antioxidants neutralize the free radicals generated by these carcinogens and thereby can reduce the risk of cancer.

Antioxidants regulate gene expression
and/or activity in cancer cells

Many studies now indicate that certain antioxidants can regulate (increase or decrease) the expression and/or activities of cellular genes, tumor-suppressor genes, and oncogenes in tumor cells in culture. Some effects of antioxidants on cell differentiation and growth inhibition in tumor cells may be related to alterations in gene expression. Changes in gene expression are seen as early as fifteen minutes after treatment with vitamin E succinate. Tables 6.1 and 6.2 list the changes in gene expression and/or activity in tumor cells in culture. The fact that antioxidants can inhibit the expression of mutated tumor-suppressor genes suggests a genetic basis for the preventive action of antioxidants. Antioxidants enhance the expression of normal tumor-suppressor genes, further suggesting the genetic basis for their action in cancer prevention. Similarly, the fact that antioxidants reduce the expression of oncogenes is also relevant to the cancer-prevention action of these antioxidants.

TABLE 6.1. THE EFFECTS OF VITAMIN E SUCCINATE ON GENE EXPRESSION AND/OR ACTIVITY IN TUMOR CELLS

Reduced Gene Expression and/or Activity	Increased Gene Expression and/or Activity
Mutated p21	Normal p21
Mutated p53	Normal p53
c-myc	TGF-beta
N-myc	Protein kinase A activity
H-ras	NA
VEGF	NA
Protein kinase C activity	NA

P21 and p53 are tumor-suppressor genes; c-myc, N-myc, and H-ras are oncogenes; VEGF (vascular endothelial growth factor) and TGF-beta (transforming growth factor-beta) are cellular genes. The levels of mRNAs of these genes represent expression. Protein kinase C and protein kinase A are enzymes and expressed as enzyme activity.

NA = not available

From K. N. Prasad and K. Che Prasad, *Fight Cancer with Vitamins and Supplements: A Guide to Prevention and Treatment,* Rochester, Vt.: Healing Arts Press, 2001.

TABLE 6.2. THE EFFECTS OF RETINOIDS AND BETA-CAROTENE ON GENE EXPRESSION AND/OR ACTIVITY IN TUMOR CELLS

Reduced Gene Expression and/or Activity	Increased Gene Expression and/or Activity
Mutated p53	Normal p53
c-myc	c-fos
c-neu	HSP70
c-erb-beta2	HSP90
H-ras	c-jun
Phosphotyrosine kinase activity	Cyclin A and D and their kinases activities
NA	MAP kinase
N/A	Connexin gene

P53 is a tumor-suppressor gene; c-myc, c-neu, c-erb-beta2, and H-ras are oncogenes; c-fos, c-jun, HSP (heat shock protein) 70 and HSP90, and cyclin A and D are cellular genes. The levels of mRNAs of these genes represent expression. Phosphotyrosine kinase and MAP kinases are enzymes and expressed as enzyme activity.

NA = not available

From K. N. Prasad and K. Che Prasad, *Fight Cancer with Vitamins and Supplements: A Guide to Prevention and Treatment,* Rochester, Vt.: Healing Arts Press, 2001.

Beta-carotene increases the expression of the connexin gene, which makes a gap-junction protein that is responsible for maintaining the link between two normal cells. Cancer cells are found to have diminished activity of the connexin gene. Retinoids and other antioxidants do not produce this effect, suggesting that it may be unique to beta-carotene. The high level of expression of the connexin gene may be one of the explanations for beta-carotene-induced cancer prevention in mammalian cells in culture. This emphasizes the importance of adding beta-carotene, together with vitamin A, to a multiple-micronutrient preparation. Unfortunately, there is serious resistance from the medical establishment for using beta-carotene in any multiple-vitamin preparation, primarily because of results of a clinical study in which synthetic beta-carotene alone increased the incidence of lung cancer in heavy tobacco smokers.

ANTIOXIDANTS STIMULATE
THE HOST'S IMMUNE SYSTEM

Although the host's immune system may not play a direct role in cancer formation, it could have an important role in rejecting newly formed cancer cells. Cancer cells are considered by the immune system to be foreign cells. An optimally functioning immune system can recognize newly formed cancer cells and kill them. A weak immune system may allow the establishment of these cancer cells, which can then grow and metastasize to distant organs in the body. Vitamins A, C, and E and beta-carotene at high but nontoxic doses enhance immune function and thereby have the potential to reduce the risk of cancer.

The studies discussed here show that the effects of antioxidants at the cellular and genetic levels are very complex and that some are directly relevant to cancer prevention. Therefore, the use of antioxidants for cancer prevention in humans has a sound scientific basis. Some cancer-preventive actions of antioxidants are summarized in Table 6.3.

TABLE 6.3. SUMMARY OF THE ACTIONS OF ANTIOXIDANTS AND SELENIUM IN CANCER PREVENTION

Antioxidants	Preventive action
Vitamin C and vitamin E	Block the formation of cancer-causing agents in the gastrointestinal tract
Most antioxidants	Block the conversion of some cancer-causing agents to active forms in the liver
Beta-carotene; vitamins A, C, and E; and selenium	Block the action of tumor-causing agents (tumor initiators and tumor promoters)
Beta-carotene; vitamins A, C, and E	Reverse newly formed or established cancer cells
Beta-carotene; vitamins A, C, and E; and selenium	Kill newly formed cancer cells in the body by stimulating the body's immune system

From K. N. Prasad and K. Che Prasad, *Fight Cancer with Vitamins and Supplements: A Guide to Prevention and Treatment*, Rochester, Vt.: Healing Arts Press, 2001.

GUIDELINES FOR SELECTING A MICRONUTRIENT PREPARATION

Cautions

The sale of micronutrient supplements totals more than $24 billion a year in the United States. If you have visited any health food store, the number of micronutrient preparations on the shelf is overwhelming. If people are not sure about what to buy, they generally rely on the advice of a salesperson at the store, who may not be very familiar with the science of micronutrients. Many rely on what they have read in popular health magazines or newspapers, or what they have been told by the representatives of the vitamin companies.

In recent years many nutrition books have been published, and some contain erroneous information regarding doses and dose schedule for supplementary micronutrients. Some nutrition books have made several misleading claims of the benefit of certain individual micronutrients. It is important to select a book based on scientific facts. Make sure that the credentials of the authors include research and teaching expertise in the area of micronutrients and cancer.

Be cautious about advice suggested in commercial advertisements through TV, radio, newspapers, magazines, or health food personnel. They can be misleading. Select your micronutrient preparation based on your age, gender, and health conditions, and check with a physician or health professional who is knowledgeable in the area of nutrition and cancer. Do not buy any vitamins or nutrients that are not fully described on the label. An independent analysis of ten randomly collected multivitamin preparations revealed that most did not have the amounts of each ingredient listed on the label. This suggests that many multivitamin preparations lack quality control. Therefore, it is important to buy nutritional products from companies that have a good reputation for this.

In multiple-vitamin preparations, certain ingredients are added without any scientific rationale. For example, inositol and choline, very important chemicals for maintaining normal function of the cells, especially nerve cells, are commonly added in amounts of 30 to 100 mg.

Because these chemicals are consumed through diet in the amount 600 to 1,000 mg, the addition of such a small amount of inositol or choline can be considered unnecessary with no health benefits. Similar statements can be made with respect to methionine.

High doses (in milligrams) of lycopene and lutein are considered important for the health of the prostate gland and eyes, respectively. In some multiple-vitamin preparations, the doses added are in micrograms (more than a thousand times less than needed for optimal benefit to the prostate gland and eyes). Again, the addition of such a small amount of lycopene and/or lutein in a multiple-vitamin preparation is unnecessary and will have no benefit to the prostate gland or eyes.

Make sure the multivitamin preparations have no iron, copper, manganese, or heavy metals such as molybdenum and zirconium. Also, do not take excessive amounts of micronutrients. Some books have suggested that one should increase the doses of a nutrient until side effects or illness become evident and then gradually decrease the doses until a comfortable level is reached. This method of selecting appropriate doses is very dangerous, because some nutrients in large amounts can cause irreversible damage.

If you have further questions consult experts who are actively involved in research, teaching, and/or patient care using micronutrients. We recommend that that you consult the scientists of Premier Micronutrient Corporation at www.mypmcinside.com, or call 615-234-4020 to discuss a micronutrient preparation for your particular need. Do research to find qualified health care professionals who can provide useful information regarding these supplements. These considerations will make your efforts to improve your health and reduce the risk of cancer more effective and less expensive.

RECOMMENDATIONS FOR A MICRONUTRIENT PREPARATION

Multiple-micronutrient preparations for cancer prevention can be developed separately for two different populations: (a) cancer-free individuals of all ages and genders with no known inherited risk of cancer, and (b) cancer-free persons who are at higher risk of developing cancer, such as heavy smokers, individuals with a family history of cancer, and cancer survivors.

The recommendations for reducing the exposure to potential carcinogens and tumor promoters in the environment, increasing fruit and vegetable intake in the diet, and adopting a healthy lifestyle are the same for both populations; however, the recommendations of micronutrient supplement are different with respect to doses and types of antioxidants. The micronutrient preparations recommended below are available commercially.

Recommendations for Micronutrient Preparations for Cancer-Free Individuals with No Known Risk of Cancer

Micronutrient formulations for cancer prevention should include dietary (vitamins A, C, and E, natural mixed carotenoids, and selenium) and endogenous antioxidants (alpha-lipoic acid and n-acetylcysteine, glutathione-elevating agents, L-carnitine, and coenzyme Q10), vitamin D elemental calcium and magnesium, B vitamins, and zinc. The proposed micronutrient preparation should not contain iron, copper, manganese, or heavy metals. It also should not contain any herbal, fruit, or vegetable antioxidants, because they do not produce unique effects that cannot be obtained by the micronutrient preparations.

The doses of micronutrients for a normal population depend on age and gender. For example, supplements for people between the ages of five and seventeen years would not contain endogenous antioxidants, because younger individuals maintain the optimal capacity for making them. Endogenous antioxidants would be included for people eighteen years and older but will be lower for those eighteen to thirty-five years than for those thirty-six years and older. Calcium and vitamin D supplementation at high doses would be included for women after the age of thirty-five. Individuals can start micronutrient supplements at any time and continue them throughout their life, in consultation with their doctors.

Recommendations for Micronutrient
Preparations for Cancer-Free High-Risk Individuals

As previously mentioned, high-risk individuals include heavy tobacco smokers, cancer survivors, or people who have a family history of cancer.

Smokers. Tobacco smoking contributes to about one-third of all cancers. At present there is no preventive strategy involving micronutrient supplementation for this population. Supplementation with a multiple-micronutrient preparation containing dietary and endogenous antioxidants, such as that proposed for nonsmokers thirty-six years or older, may reduce the health-associated risks of smoking, including cancer. Smokers can start the micronutrient supplementation at any time and continue throughout their life, in consultation with their doctor.

Individuals with a family history of cancer. Individuals with a family history of cancer may consider taking micronutrient preparations earlier in life—perhaps as early as five years—and continue for their entire life. Many have presumed that the genetic basis of cancer cannot be delayed or prevented, but a recent laboratory study suggests that multiple micronutrients may help. The study of the effect of a mixture of dietary and endogenous antioxidants on proton radiation–induced cancer in *Drosophila melanogaster* (fruit flies) suggests that antioxidants can reduce the incidence of genetically based cancer. For example, female fruit flies carrying the mutant HOP (TUM-1) gene become very sensitive to developing a leukemia-like cancer. Exposure to proton radiation markedly enhances the incidence of this cancer. Supplementation with an antioxidant mixture before and after irradiation completely blocks the radiation-induced cancer (Prasad, in collaboration with Dr. Sharmila Bhattacharya of NASA, at Moffett Field, Calif.). This result obtained from fruit flies cannot be extrapolated to humans, but it suggests that antioxidants have the potential to reduce the risk or delay the appearance of tumors in individuals with a family history of cancer.

These individuals should take a micronutrient preparation similar to that for normal people age thirty-six or older, described above. As previously mentioned, they can start micronutrient supplemention at any time and continue it throughout their life, in consultation with their doctors.

Cancer survivors. Increased numbers of cancer patients are surviving because of advancement in cancer therapy (surgery, chemotherapy, and radiation therapy). However, they exhibit short- and long-term adverse health effects induced by the cancer-treatment agents. Short-term effects include memory impairment, fatigue, peripheral neuropathy, and increased susceptibility to infection because of impaired immune function. Some of these symptoms can last for a long time. Long-term adverse health effects include the recurrence of initial primary tumors and the development of secondary new tumors. A proposed micronutrient preparation for this population would be the same as that for other high-risk groups, such as smokers.

Based on the results of scientific studies, supplementation with multiple micronutrients containing dietary and endogenous antioxidants will reduce the risk of recurrence of primary tumors as well as the appearance of new tumors that are induced by treatment agents. This formulation can be started a week after completion of standard therapy and be continued throughout one's life, after consultation with a doctor.

TAMOXIFEN AND MICRONUTRIENTS IN BREAST-CANCER PREVENTION

Populations at higher risk of developing breast cancer include women over the age of sixty, and women with a family history of breast cancer or who carry a mutated form of breast-cancer genes (BRCA1 and BRCA2). In the Breast Cancer Prevention Trial, women who received tamoxifen, an antiestrogen agent, had a lower incidence of breast cancer than women who did not receive the drug. In the Study of Tamoxifen and Raloxifene, researchers observed that both drugs were equally effective in reducing the incidence of breast cancer in postmenopausal women who are at increased risk of developing this disease.

The adverse effects of tamoxifen include bone loss in premenopausal women and development of hyperlipidemia (increased levels of lipids, such as cholesterol, in the blood), which increases the risk of stroke in some women. A clinical study has reported that supplementation with a mixture of vitamins C and E reduces the onset of hyperlipidemia. Thus, a combination of tamoxifen and a micronutrient preparation recommended for individuals over the age of thirty-six may reduce the side effects of tamoxifen without reducing its effectiveness.

RATIONALE FOR USING MULTIPLE MICRONUTRIENTS IN PROPOSED CANCER-PREVENTIVE STRATEGY

Multiple micronutrients including dietary and endogenous antioxidants are recommended, because many different types of free radicals are produced. Each antioxidant has a different affinity for each of these free radicals, depending on the cellular environment, and they are distributed differently in organs and within the same cells. The gradient of oxygen pressure varies within the cell and tissues. Vitamin E is more effective as a quencher of free radicals in reduced oxygen pressure, whereas beta-carotene and vitamin A are more effective at higher oxygen pressure.

Vitamin C is necessary to protect cellular components in aqueous environments, whereas carotenoids, vitamin A, and vitamin E protect cellular components in lipid (fatty) environments. Vitamin C also plays an important role in maintaining cellular levels of vitamin E by recycling the vitamin E radical (oxidized) to the reduced (antioxidant) form. Also, the DNA damage produced by oxidized vitamin C can be decreased by vitamin E. The form and type of vitamin E used in a micronutrient preparation is also important to improve its beneficial effects. For example, various organs of rats selectively accumulate the most effective form of vitamin E, otherwise known as the natural form or alpha-tocopheryl succinate (vitamin E succinate). We have reported that oral ingestion of vitamin E succinate (800 IU per day) for over six months increased plasma levels in humans not only of alpha-tocopherol but also of vitamin E succinate, suggesting that vitamin E succinate can be absorbed from the intestinal tract without hydrolysis to alpha-tocopherol, provided the body store of alpha-tocopherol is full.

Selenium, a cofactor of glutathione peroxidase, acts as an antioxidant. Therefore, selenium supplementation together with other dietary and endogenous antioxidants is also essential.

Glutathione, one of the endogenously made compounds, represents a potent intracellular protective agent against oxidative damage. It destroys hydrogen peroxide (H_2O_2) and anions and is very effective in quenching peroxynitrite. Therefore, increasing the intracellular levels of glutathione is essential for the protection of various organelles within the cells. Oral supplementation with glutathione failed to significantly increase plasma levels of glutathione in human subjects, suggesting that this tripeptide is completely destroyed in the gastrointestinal (GI) tract. N-acetylcysteine and alpha-lipoic acid, which are absorbed by the GI tract, increase the intracellular levels of glutathione and, therefore, can be used in combination with dietary antioxidants.

Coenzyme Q10 is needed by the mitochondria to generate energy. In addition, it also scavenges peroxy radicals faster than alpha-tocopherol and, like, vitamin C, can regenerate vitamin E in a redox cycle (converting the oxidized form of vitamin E to the reduced form that acts as an antioxidant).

UNIQUE FEATURES OF THE PROPOSED MICRONUTRIENT PREPARATION

The proposed micronutrient formulations do not contain iron, copper, or manganese, because these trace minerals are known to combine with vitamin C to produce free radicals that could reduce optimal effects. In addition, these trace minerals in the presence of antioxidants are absorbed more efficiently by the body and could increase the body stores of free forms of the minerals. Increased body stores of free iron and copper have been associated with the enhanced risk of many chronic human diseases, including cancer.

All proposed micronutrient preparations should contain both vitamin A and natural mixed carotenoids (90 percent beta-carotene). This is because beta-carotene, in addition to acting as a precursor of vitamin A, performs unique functions that cannot be produced by vitamin A, and vice versa. As stated previously, beta-carotene increases the expression of the connexin gene, which codes for a gap-junction protein that holds two normal cells together, whereas vitamin A does not. Vitamin A produces differentiation in normal cells during development as well as in cancer cells, but beta-carotene does not. Beta-carotene is more effective in quenching oxygen radicals than most other antioxidants.

All micronutrient formulations should contain two forms of vitamin E: d-alpha-tocopheryl acetate and d-alpha-tocopheryl succinate (vitamin E succinate). Vitamin E succinate is now considered the most effective form of vitamin E, because it is more soluble than alpha-tocopherol and it more easily enters the cells, where it is converted to alpha-tocopherol and thus provides intracellular protection against oxidative damage. Vitamin E succinate can also produce some unique biological effects that cannot be produced by alpha-tocopherol. Therefore, in order to increase efficacy, both forms of vitamin E are essential.

As stated earlier, micronutrient supplements should be taken orally in two doses, half in the morning and the other half in the evening with a meal. This is because the biological half-lives of micronutrients are highly variable and can create fluctuations in micronutrient levels in the tissue. A twofold difference in the levels of certain antioxidants, such as vitamin E succinate, can cause a marked difference in the expression of gene profiles (Prasad, unpublished).

A well-designed clinical trial using the proposed preventive strategy should be initiated in a high-risk cancer-free population as well as in cancer survivors. In the meantime, individuals in high-risk populations may choose to adopt the proposed cancer prevention strategy in consultation with their physicians.

Reducing exposure to potential carcinogens from diet, environment, and lifestyle appears to be the most effective strategy for reducing the risk of cancer in humans; however, it is the most difficult strategy to implement. X-rays are commonly used to detect and diagnose disease and, therefore, should not be avoided when necessary. Avoiding ultraviolet radiation from sun exposure is perhaps the easiest of all cancer-preventive strategies, but in the summer the beaches are full of sunbathers. Because of the addictive nature of tobacco smoking, and in spite of major educational programs and state and federal laws prohibiting smoking in public places, there has been no significant change in the number of smokers in the United States.

Dietary habits are difficult to alter. Human diets contain both cancer-protective substances and cancer-causing agents (mutagens and carcinogens). Most of the mutagenic and carcinogenic substances that are present in the diet occur naturally; however, small amounts have been introduced into the diet by the use of pesticides in agriculture production. These issues are usually beyond our control, with the exception of exclusively consuming certified organic produce. Mutagens are formed during cooking; the browning of vegetables or meat during cooking is an indication of mutagen formation. Flame-broiled fatty meat contains much higher levels of carcinogens, such as benzo(a)pyrene, than those found in oven-cooked meat. The dietary recommendation to eat fresh fruits and vegetables, limit intake of fat, and increase intake of fiber are difficult to implement consistently over a long period of time.

INTERVENTIONAL TRIALS
WITH MULTIPLE ANTIOXIDANTS

Some clinical trials in which multiple dietary antioxidants were used support our theory that using multiple micronutrients containing dietary and endogenous antioxidants helps to reduce the risk of cancer. Some of these studies are described below.

Oral administration of multiple micronutrients including high doses of dietary antioxidants and bacille bilie de Calmette-Guérin (BCG) vaccine, which is known to stimulate immune function, lowered the rate of recurrence of human bladder cancer by 40 percent in five years, compared with a daily multivitamin supplement containing antioxidants at recommended daily levels (see Table 6.4). This is an impressive and promising result, even though no endogenous antioxidants and no diet or lifestyle changes were included. In this study the dose of vitamin A was very high and could produce liver and skin toxicity after long-term consumption. In addition, the vitamin B_6 dose was also very high and could cause peripheral neuropathy. The addition of endogenous antioxidants, and a diet low in fat and high in fiber, would likely have improved the efficacy of this micronutrient regimen without requiring the high doses of vitamins A and B_6.

TABLE 6.4. EFFECT OF HIGH-DOSE MULTIPLE DIETARY ANTIOXIDANTS ON THE RECURRENCE OF HUMAN BLADDER CANCER

Micronutrients per day	Recurrence of bladder cancer
EXPERIMENTAL GROUP	
Vitamin A, 40,000 IU	
Vitamin C, 2,000 mg	
Vitamin E, 400 IU	
Vitamin B_6, 100 mg	40 percent
A multiple vitamin containing RDA value of each nutrient	
BCG vaccine	
CONTROL GROUP	
A multiple vitamin containing RDA value of each nutrient	80 percent

From K. N. Prasad and K. C. Prasad, *Fight Cancer with Vitamins and Supplements: A Guide to Prevention and Treatment,* Rochester, Vt.: Healing Arts Press, 2001.

Another study, which was performed in a rural hospital in Italy, showed that daily oral consumption of a mixture of high-dose multiple dietary antioxidants reduced the recurrence of colon polyps (adenomas) by about 30 percent. Daily intake of a large amount of fiber (cellulose) also minimized the recurrence of colon polyps by 21 percent (see Table 6.5). It remains to be established whether a combination of multiple micronutrients including dietary and endogenous antioxidants with a diet low in fat and high in fiber, in addition to changes in lifestyle, would produce more impressive results.

TABLE 6.5. EFFECT OF SEVERAL HIGH-DOSE DIETARY ANTIOXIDANTS OR HIGH FIBER ON THE RECURRENCE OF COLON POLYPS AMONG RURAL ITALIANS

Micronutrients per day	Reduction in recurrence of colon polyps
EXPERIMENTAL GROUP	
Vitamin A, 3,000 IU	
Vitamin C, 1,000 milligrams	30 percent
Vitamin E, 70 milligrams	
CONTROL GROUP—NO VITAMIN SUPPLEMENT	

From K. N. Prasad and K. C. Prasad, *Fight Cancer with Vitamins and Supplements: A Guide to Prevention and Treatment,* Rochester, Vt.: Healing Arts Press, 2001.

In contrast to the studies mentioned above, a U.S. investigation reported no beneficial effects of high-dose multiple dietary antioxidants on the recurrence of colon polyps. This study utilized the following antioxidants per day: synthetic beta-carotene, 25 mg; vitamin C, 1,000 mg; and vitamin E, 400 mg. Another U.S. study failed to report the beneficial effects of high-dose fiber alone on the recurrence of colon polyps.

These interventional trials, which examined the effects of multiple dietary antioxidants on the recurrence of colon polyps, are difficult to compare. The Italian study used vitamin A, whereas as the U.S. study used synthetic beta-carotene. Synthetic beta-carotene has been found to be inactive in some biological systems (such as radiation-induced cancer formation). In addition, some preparations of synthetic beta-carotene reportedly have no beta-carotene activity. The U.S. study did not measure the purity of its synthetic beta-carotene. For optimal effect, both natural beta-carotene and vitamin A should have been used. No modifications in diet or lifestyle were recommended in either study. It is reasonable to assume that patients in the rural Italian hospital had a lower-fat diet compared with patients in the United States.

The value of high fiber in combination with multiple antioxidants is underscored by another U.S. study, which reported that vitamin C (4,000 mg per day) and vitamin E (400 mg per day), in combination with a high-fiber diet of more than 12 g per day for a period of four years, reduced the recurrence of colon polyps more than the same dose of antioxidants without large amounts of fiber. The addition of other dietary antioxidants and endogenous antioxidants and a low-fat diet might have produced more impressive results.

A joint U.S. and Chinese study found that high-dose (two to three times the RDA value of each nutrient) multiple micronutrients (synthetic beta-carotene, synthetic vitamin E, and selenium) reduced mortality by 10 percent and cancer incidence by 13 percent in high-risk populations. This study did not recommend diet or lifestyle changes or the consumption of endogenous antioxidants.

In some cases very high doses of individual antioxidants have produced beneficial effects on the recurrence of primary tumors. For example, vitamin A supplementation at a dose of 300,000 IU per day for 12 months reduced the recurrence of primary nonsmall-cell lung carcinoma (a form of lung cancer) by 11 percent. This high a dose of vitamin A, however, cannot be taken over a long period of time because of toxicity.

High doses of beta-carotene, retinoids, and synthetic vitamin E alone or in combination can cause varying degrees of regression of oral leukoplakia, a potentially precancerous lesion of the oral cavity. Studies on this topic were conducted for a short period of time. The recommended cancer-prevention steps for high-risk populations may be more effective in causing regression of oral leukoplakia than the individual antioxidants.

ADDITIONAL BENEFITS OF FOLLOWING CANCER-PREVENTION GUIDELINES

The benefits of changing one's diet, taking supplementary micronutrients, and changing one's lifestyle is not limited to cancer protection—they also help in healthy aging. Increased oxidative damage and chronic inflammation are involved in the progression of aging, but antioxidants are known to reduce oxidative damage and chronic inflammation. Following the guidelines of cancer prevention may also help in reducing the risk of chronic illnesses such as heart disease, Alzheimer's disease, Parkinson's disease, and diabetes, all of which are characterized by increased oxidative damage and chronic inflammation. Since antioxidants reduce oxidative damage and inhibit chronic inflammation, the use of the same micronutrient preparation may also reduce the risk of other chronic diseases.

CONCLUDING REMARKS

Most epidemiologic studies suggest that a diet low in fat and high in fiber (from fruits, vegetables, and high-fiber cereals) may reduce the risk of cancer. However, clinical studies on high-fiber diets alone or low-fat diets alone have produced inconsistent results on cancer risk, from no effect to beneficial effects. Other survey-type studies suggested that a diet rich in antioxidants may reduce the risk of cancer, but the clinical studies with the individual antioxidants produced similarly inconsistent results. We believe that supplementation with a multiple-micronutrient preparation containing dietary and endogenous antioxidants, in addition to changes in the diet and lifestyle, are equally important and may lower the risk of cancers in humans. These three factors are equally important in cancer prevention.

Based on laboratory and human studies, we have proposed guidelines for selecting a multiple-micronutrient preparation appropriate for one's age, gender, and health conditions. We have also suggested adopting changes in diet and lifestyle for cancer prevention. Although the guidelines for the diet and lifestyle are not expected to change in the near future, the dose and type of micronutrients in the multivitamin preparation will be changed whenever new scientific data become available. (For example, based on new scientific data, we have proposed a reduction in the dose of vitamin A from 5,000 IU to 3,000 IU per day, and an increase in vitamin D_3 from 400 IU to 800 IU.)

8 Micronutrients in Combination with Radiation Therapy, Chemotherapy, and Experimental Therapies

CANCER MORTALITY

As already stated, the U.S. mortality rate from cancer has not changed significantly during the past several decades in spite of extensive research and development of new treatment modalities. Cancer patients can be divided into three groups: (1) those who receive standard therapy (radiation and/or chemotherapy) or experimental therapies (heat therapy, immunotherapy, or gene therapy), (2) those who become unresponsive to these therapies, and (3) those in remission (survivors). There are few effective methods of reducing the toxicity of chemotherapy or radiation therapy. Also, there is no effective strategy to prolong the life span, with a good quality of life, in patients who become unresponsive to all standard and experimental therapies. Except for reducing the risk of recurrence of breast cancer with low-dose tamoxifen, there is no effective strategy to reduce the risk of recurrence of the primary tumor or the development of second new cancers induced by treatment agents.

Standard cancer therapy has reached a plateau in treating most solid tumors—despite impressive progress in radiation therapy, such as dosimetry, and more efficient methods of delivery of radiation to tumors. The effectiveness of chemotherapy, which involves the use of multiple drugs with different modes of action, has also reached a plateau. Therefore, additional approaches should be developed to improve the efficacy of standard therapy, to reduce the risk of recurrence of primary tumors and the development of second new cancers, and to improve the quality of life of those patients who become unresponsive to all therapies.

WHAT IS THE CURRENT STATUS OF CANCER THERAPY?

Before discussing the role of multiple micronutrients in combination with radiation therapy, chemotherapy, or experimental therapy, we will outline the nature of cancer cells and the present status, usefulness, and limitations of standard forms of therapy.

Are All Cells of a Particular Cancer Similar?

If all cells of a specific type of cancer were similar, treating cancer would be easier, because one therapeutic agent would kill all the cancer cells. Unfortunately, cancer cells are very complex; there are many different kinds, even within the same tumor, and they differ in sensitivity to chemotherapy, radiation, and experimental therapy. Therefore, multiple drugs—known as chemotherapeutic agents—are typically used in treating tumors.

Cancer cells may become unresponsive to all therapeutic agents, including drugs, radiation, and experimental therapeutic agents, after a period of good initial response (tumor regression). During treatment these agents can produce several biochemical and genetic changes among the cancer cells that are not killed, creating "super" cancer cells that become very resistant. Such cells may become sensitive to entirely different groups of treatment agents, such as heat therapy, immunotherapy, or high-dose antioxidants, which kill cancer cells through mechanisms that are totally different from those produced by chemotherapeutic agents or radiation. In addition, they would ideally kill cancer cells without killing normal cells.

BENEFITS AND LIMITATIONS OF VARIOUS CANCER TREATMENTS

Current standard cancer therapies include surgery, chemotherapy, and radiation therapy, whereas experimental therapies include hyperthermia (heat therapy), immunotherapy, and gene therapy. Frequently, surgery is performed first, followed by chemotherapy and/or radiation therapy. Generally, experimental therapies are used when tumor cells are not responding to chemotherapy or radiation therapy. The usefulness and limitations of each of these therapeutic agents are discussed here.

Standard Cancer Therapy

Surgery

Surgery is one of the most common procedures in the treatment of solid tumors. Potentially precancerous lesions, such as atypical moles that could become malignant melanoma or colon polyps that have a chance of becoming colon cancer, are removed surgically. When surgery is done to remove cancer, some cancer cells are often left in the body and can be later treated by chemotherapy and/or radiation therapy. Nevertheless, surgery is considered one of the best available approaches to treat solid tumors because it does not increase the risk of new cancers or noncancerous diseases among survivors. The use of therapeutic doses of multiple micronutrients containing dietary and endogenous antioxidants, in combination with a balanced diet rich in fruits and vegetables, may help patients recover from surgery faster.

Chemotherapy

Several toxic drugs are used extensively in treating cancer, frequently in combination with surgery and/or radiation therapy. Almost all of them kill both cancer cells and normal cells and, therefore, cannot be considered ideal for treating cancer. However, chemotherapy has been useful in increasing the survival rates or times of patients with certain tumors, such as Hodgkin's lymphoma, childhood leukemia, and testicular cancer.

Chemotherapy causes severe illness, impairs the body's immune system, and increases the risk of new cancers among patients who survive more than five years after treatment. In some instances severe damage to normal tissue becomes the limiting factor for the continuation of therapy. Chemotherapy is not as effective for the treatment of melanoma, brain tumors, and lung cancer as compared to other types of cancer.

Reports show that the incidence of leukemia (blood cancer) and solid tumors among survivors of chemotherapy and radiation therapy is about 10 percent, but the observation period on which this figure is based is usually no more than ten years after the completion of treatment. According to present knowledge, the risk of leukemia may not increase ten years after treatment, but the risk of solid cancers and noncancerous diseases, such as aplastic anemia and developmental delay in children, persists for up to thirty years or more after treatment. Therefore, additional approaches must be developed to improve the efficacy of chemotherapy and may involve the use of nontoxic agents, such as therapeutic doses of dietary antioxidants that can protect normal cells without protecting cancer cells. In spite of these limitations, chemotherapy must be used until better treatment methods are established.

Radiation Therapy

Radiation in the form of X-rays or gamma rays is a typical treatment method for many types of human cancer. Occasionally neutron radiation or proton radiation is used. The advantage of these is that they can kill cancer cells that are normally resistant to X-ray irradiation or gamma irradiation. The disadvantage of neutron radiation and proton radiation is that they are more damaging to normal cells than X-rays or gamma rays. Radiation therapy is frequently used in combination with surgery or chemotherapy or both. Some cancers, such as childhood leukemia, Hodgkin's lymphoma, testicular embryonal carcinoma, and neuroblastoma, respond to radiation therapy very well, whereas other cancers, such as melanoma, respond very poorly.

Like chemotherapy, radiation therapy has toxic effects. It kills both normal and cancer cells, causes severe illness, impairs the body's defense system, and increases the risk of new cancer among those who survive. In some instances severe damage to normal tissue becomes the limiting factor for the continuation of the therapy. Generally, the time interval between radiation exposure and detection of new tumors is three to ten years for leukemia and up to thirty years or more for solid tumors. The risk of noncancerous diseases, such as aplastic anemia or delayed necrosis (a form of ulcer that is difficult to heal) in organs containing cells that normally do not divide (such as the brain and liver), also persists after completion of treatment. In spite of these limitations, radiation therapy must be used until better treatment methods are established. The use of nontoxic agents, such as therapeutic doses of dietary antioxidants that can protect normal cells without protecting cancer cells against radiation damage, or agents that can increase the effect of irradiation on cancer cells but not on normal cells, would improve the efficacy of radiation treatment.

Experimental Cancer Therapies

Hyperthermia (Heat Therapy)

Tumor cells are more sensitive to heat than normal cells with respect to cell death and growth inhibition. Heat therapy was discovered accidentally in 1893, when cancer patients of Dr. William Coley of Columbia University, New York, experienced high fevers due to infection. Since antibiotics had not yet been discovered, these fevers persisted for a few days. Dr. Coley observed that some of the tumors of patients with fevers shrank markedly. This remarkable discovery remained relatively obscure until the 1960s, when radiation biologists reinvestigated heat therapy. At present, temperatures of 42 to 43°C (107.6 to 109.4°F) are commonly used in heat therapy, primarily for the purpose of controlling local tumors. Heat therapy is given when all standard therapies have failed. However, sometimes heat is used in combination with radiation therapy. This approach has provided occasional local relief for some cancer patients with localized tumors. The results of heat therapy, thus far, have been disappointing.

In the case of tumors that have spread, whole-body heat therapy would be more desirable than localized heat therapy. Raising the whole-body temperature from 37°C (98.6°F) to 42°C or 43°C, even for a short time, can cause severe adverse effects. Some laboratory experiments suggest that the use of such high temperatures in combination with radiation actually may increase the risk of radiation-induced cancer. Because of this, the use of high temperatures cannot be considered in designing long-term heat-treatment strategies for human cancer. Whole-body heat therapy at a lower temperature (40°C, or 104°F), in combination with nontoxic chemicals that increase the effect of heat, may be of value in treating human cancer, because the whole-body temperature can be raised from 37°C to 40°C for a short period of time without toxic effects. Heat therapy could be given at the beginning rather than at the end of standard therapy to help reduce tumor size before treatment. This makes it possible for the amounts of chemotherapeutic agents or radiation to be reduced.

Immunotherapy

Antibodies are also called immunoglobulins (Igs). They are gamma-globulin proteins present in the circulating blood. The immune system uses them to identify and neutralize foreign agents, such as bacteria and viruses. Antibodies to specific cellular proteins are produced by biotechnology companies with the assumption that they will help kill cancer cells that bind to these antibodies. Unfortunately, the antibodies are not specific for cancer cells; they also can bind with many normal cells. Thus, their usefulness in treating cancer is limited. Antibodies obtained from the heat-shock protein (proteins that are produced in response to high temperatures or physical stress and are normally present in both cancer cells and normal cells) of tumor cells selectively kill tumor cells without affecting normal cells. Such antibodies have produced some beneficial effects on certain tumors but have not been widely accepted as a method of cancer treatment. Certain types of bacteria, and even a patient's own tumor cells, are inactivated for use in immunotherapy. Varying degrees of tumor regression have been observed with these treatments.

In addition, attempts have been made through genetic engineering to make a preparation of the patient's own natural killer cells that are more efficient at killing tumor cells. Such immunotherapy has caused varying degrees of tumor regression. Dendritic cells are known to stimulate immune function that can kill cancer cells without affecting normal cells, and they have been used in the treatment of certain tumors with minimal success.

Gene Therapy

This involves the delivery of toxic genes to tumor cells, or drugs targeting mutated genes that are present only in cancer cells. Theoretically, gene therapy selectively kills cancer cells. The major limitation of this approach has been gene delivery to the target tumor tissue. The few clinical trials performed have not shown encouraging results. For this reason the role of gene therapy in the management of human tumors remains uncertain. Extensive laboratory and clinical studies on gene therapy are being conducted.

Anti-Angiogenesis Drug Therapy

This entails the use of drugs that inhibit angiogenesis, or the formation of blood vessels. As tumors grow, new blood vessels are formed in order to deliver nutrition to the tumors. Scientists once thought that an anti-angiogenesis drug would inhibit the formation of new blood vessels and thus starve the tumor to death. Indeed, anti-angiogenesis drugs have cured tumors in mice. Unfortunately, clinical trials with anti-angiogenesis drugs have not been encouraging, owing to the toxicities of the drugs. Nontoxic anti-angiogenesis drugs would cause selective tumor regression. Laboratory experiments have shown that vitamin E succinate, a nontoxic derivative of vitamin E, and n-acetylcysteine (a glutathione-elevating agent) at therapeutic doses inhibit angiogenesis. These agents could be useful in anti-angiogenesis therapy.

Sodium Butyrate and Interferon-Alpha-2b

Butyric acid, a small fatty acid, is formed in large amounts in the lower colon. This fatty acid or its analog, phenylbutyrate, have induced apoptosis (cell death) and inhibited growth of several rodent and human tumor cells in culture. Interferon-alpha-2b is produced by immune cells and has shown anticancer activity in laboratory studies. However, clinical studies with these agents produced minimal benefits. Therefore, any nontoxic agent that can enhance the cell-killing effect of sodium butyrate, phenylbutyrate, or interferon-alpha-2b would enhance the value of these agents in clinical studies. Laboratory experiments show that vitamin E succinate increases the growth-inhibiting effects of sodium butyrate and interferon-alpha-2b on cancer cells.

Delayed Health Consequences of Standard Cancer Therapies

The treatment methods available at the present have produced a growing number of long-term survivors of early stage cancers such as Hodgkin's lymphoma, childhood leukemia, Wilms' tumor (kidney cancer), cervical cancer, prostate cancer, neuroblastoma, and retinoblastoma. There is a risk that new cancers and noncancerous diseases will develop in these patients. In addition, the risk of recurrence of the primary tumors exists.

Based on five-year survival rates, significant progress has been made in the treatment of some cancers. But if one considers the fact that there is a growing risk of new cancers and noncancerous diseases, a concern is raised about the consequences and adequacy of available methods of treatment. Noncancerous diseases that may afflict survivors include:

1. Aplastic anemia (due to damage to bone-marrow cells that produce red blood cells), if the bone marrow was targeted by therapy
2. Paralysis, if the spinal cord was involved in radiation therapy
3. Cataracts, if one or both eyes were affected by radiation therapy

4. Reproductive failure, if reproductive organs were involved in therapy

5. Necrosis (a form of tissue destruction) in organs in which the cells don't divide, such as the brain and muscles, if they were affected by radiation therapy

6. Retardation of growth, if the patients were children

7. Cognitive problems, if the brains of children were involved in therapy

Because of these potential risks, newer approaches to cancer treatments that utilize nontoxic agents, which reduce the toxicity of chemotherapy and radiation therapy, or which can enhance the cell-killing effects of these agents without affecting normal tissue, must be developed. Until better therapies are available, present methods of treatment should be continued.

Improved Methods of Cancer Treatment

The ideal way to treat cancer would be to convert all cancer cells into cells that are more like normal cells (noncancerous) or to kill all cancer cells without killing normal cells, or both. To achieve the first goal we need to understand the basic steps in maintaining the regular features of normal cells and the fundamental biological changes that convert normal cells to cancer cells. To achieve the second goal we must identify substances that kill cancer cells without killing normal cells. If one considers the evolution of cancer cells in the body it is possible to discover nontoxic agents that can change cancer cells to more normal-like cells and/or that can kill only tumor cells. Indeed, several such agents have been identified, including some high-dose antioxidants, butyric acid, and heat therapy. Unfortunately, these agents have not been investigated in humans in an appropriate manner.

The conversion from normal cells to cancer cells probably occurs more frequently than we realize. However, these newly formed cancer cells do not always develop into detectable cancer, possibly because the body has an elaborate defense, which includes the immune system and antioxidant systems. When cancer cells escape these defense systems, tumor cells can establish themselves in the host and grow. Occasionally spontaneous regression of some cancers, such as neuroblastoma, has been observed. This implies that the body has a defense system that potentially can reject and destroy even well-established tumors.

Micronutrient Therapy

Micronutrients include dietary (vitamins A, C, and E and carotenoids and selenium) and endogenous (glutathione, alpha-lipoic acid, coenzyme Q10, and L-carnitine) antioxidants, vitamin D and B vitamins, and minerals such as iron, copper, and manganese. At therapeutic doses, antioxidants such as vitamins A, C, and E and carotenoids have been shown to play a part in the process of differentiation and growth inhibition of cancer cells. They also kill cancer cells without affecting normal cells. Other micronutrients, such as B vitamins and minerals, are depleted during radiation therapy or chemotherapy. Antioxidants in combination are more effective than the individual agents in limiting the growth of cancer cells.

At present the role of antioxidants in cancer treatment is controversial, and most oncologists or radiation therapists discourage patients from taking antioxidant supplements during radiation therapy or chemotherapy. They fear that antioxidants may protect both cancer cells and normal cells against therapeutic agents and thereby reduce the effectiveness of the treatment. On the other hand, some scientists, including us, believe that there are substantial amounts of laboratory data and some human studies that suggest that antioxidants do not protect cancer cells against radiation damage, and, in fact, have potential to kill cancer cells without killing normal cells, thus increasing the effectiveness of radiation therapy. Can these opposing views be reconciled? Before we can answer this question, we should understand the reasons for the current controversies. They are:

1. Failure to distinguish between the effects of preventive and therapeutic doses of antioxidants alone or in combination with standard treatment agents on cancer cells

2. Failure to appreciate the selective killing effect of therapeutic doses of antioxidants on cancer cells but not on normal cells

3. Assuming that the effect of a single antioxidant (e.g., beta-carotene, vitamin E, or selenium) in clinical prevention or treatment studies would be similar to those produced by a multiple vitamin preparation containing therapeutic doses of antioxidants

4. Relying on data obtained from the use of a single antioxidant in prevention studies as a reason for not recommending antioxidants during treatment

PREVENTIVE AND THERAPEUTIC DOSE RANGE OF ANTIOXIDANTS IN HUMANS

In order to clarify the above issues, it is essential to define the dose range of preventive and therapeutic doses of antioxidants. Preventive doses do not affect the growth of cancer cells or normal cells, whereas therapeutic doses inhibit the growth of cancer cells without affecting the growth of normal cells.

The proposed daily *oral preventive dose* ranges of antioxidants for adults at high risk for developing cancer are as follows:

- vitamin A: up to 3,000 IU
- vitamin C: up to 2 grams
- vitamin E (alpha-tocopherol, alpha-tocopheryl acetate, or alpha-tocopheryl succinate): up to 400 IU
- carotenoids including beta-carotene: up to 25 milligrams
- selenomethionine: up to 100 micrograms (mcg)
- coenzyme Q10: up to 100 milligrams
- alpha-lipoic acid: up to 100 milligrams
- n-acetylcysteine: up to 200 milligrams
- L-carnitine: up to 200 milligrams

The doses of these antioxidants for a lower risk population would be lower than for a high-risk population. Preventive doses for children would be lower than for adults.

The proposed daily *oral therapeutic dose* ranges of antioxidants for patients undergoing standard therapy or who are unresponsive to all therapies are as follows:

- vitamin A: 10,000 IU or more
- vitamin C: 5 grams or more
- vitamin E (alpha-tocopherol, alpha-tocopheryl acetate, or alpha-tocopheryl succinate): up to 1,600 IU
- carotenoids including beta-carotene: up to 100 milligrams
- selenomethionine: up to 300 micrograms (mcg)
- coenzyme Q10: up to 400 milligrams
- alpha-lipoic acid: up to 500 milligrams
- n-acetylcysteine: up to 500 milligrams
- L-carnitine: up to 500 milligrams

Endogenous antioxidants such as alpha-lipoic acid and n-acetylcysteine that enhance glutathione levels in the cells should not be used in a multivitamin preparation to be used during chemotherapy or radiation therapy, because they may protect normal and cancer cells. However, all dietary and endogenous antioxidants will be used in patients who become unresponsive to all standard and experimental therapies. Treatment doses for children would be lower than for adults. The use of treatment doses of antioxidants will continue only during the entire period of therapy, after which, a multiple micronutrient preparation containing preventive doses of antioxidants would be used in survivors.

Recommendations and Use of Antioxidants by Patients

Most oncologists discourage patients from taking antioxidant supplements during radiation therapy, chemotherapy, or experimental therapy and even after completion of therapy, and this may prevent some patients from receiving the benefits of antioxidants. A few oncologists may recommend a multiple-vitamin preparation containing low doses (preventive doses, primarily RDA values) of antioxidants during and after therapy, but this has the potential to be harmful, as laboratory results have shown that low doses of individual dietary antioxidants may increase the growth of some cancer cells (Prasad et al. 1999; Crowe, Kim, and Chandraratna 2003; Verma et al. 2004), especially those residual primary cancer cells that may lead to the recurrence of primary tumors. Such cancerous regrowth would become detectable within a few years.

Despite the recommendations of many oncologists for not taking antioxidants during therapy, more than 60 percent of cancer patients use antioxidant supplements in one form or another, and many combine them with standard therapy without their oncologists' knowledge (Richardson et al. 2000). This may be harmful, because a low, preventive-dose multiple-vitamin preparation may interfere with the efficacy of standard therapy. Some studies have shown that low doses of antioxidants such as vitamin E, vitamin C, n-acetylcysteine, alpha-lipoic acid, selenium, retinol, or beta-carotene protected cancer cells against free-radical damage produced by chemotherapeutic agents or radiation (Prasad and Kumar 1996; Salganik 2001; Labriola and Livingston 1999; Witenberg et al. 1999; Miyajimaet al. 1999; Heaney et al. 2008).

Potential to Improve Standard or Experimental Cancer Therapy with Antioxidants

Several laboratory experiments and limited clinical studies show that individual antioxidants and their derivatives at therapeutic doses, and after a prolonged treatment period, inhibit the growth of several types of tumor cells without affecting the growth of normal cells. Laboratory studies suggest that dietary antioxidants at therapeutic doses also protect normal cells against damage produced by radiation therapy or chemotherapy without protecting cancer cells. Some laboratory experiments have revealed that these antioxidants can increase the growth-inhibiting effects of ionizing radiation and chemotherapeutic agents in a synergistic manner, thus improving the efficacy of standard therapy by reducing its toxicity and increasing tumor-cell death.

In order to effectively use antioxidants during standard therapy, it is essential to consider the following established concepts.

1. Tumor cells and cancer cells respond differently to antioxidant doses.
2. The effects of therapeutic doses of antioxidants on cancer cells are different from those produced by preventive doses of antioxidants.
3. Therapeutic doses of antioxidants not only inhibit the growth of tumor cells but also enhance the effectiveness of standard therapy while potentially reducing its toxicity.
4. Preventive doses of antioxidants may increase the growth of cancer cells and reduce the efficacy of standard therapy.
5. Multiple antioxidants are more effective than a single antioxidant.
6. Therapeutic doses of antioxidants should be administered orally twice a day three to five days before the start of radiation therapy and/or chemotherapy and continue for the entire treatment period.
7. After completion of treatment, the therapeutic doses of antioxidants should be replaced by preventive doses of antioxidants for one's entire life span.

Substantial numbers of laboratory and animal studies have been done on therapeutic doses or preventive doses of antioxidants alone or in combination with radiation or chemotherapeutic agents. See chapter 6 for our recommendations on new clinical studies to examine the use of multiple dietary antioxidants in cancer treatment. In addition, several laboratory and limited human studies suggest that therapeutic doses of antioxidants alone kill cancer cells without killing normal cells and increase the cancer-cell-killing effect of radiation or chemotherapeutic agents. These studies are described here.

Studies on the Effects of Therapeutic Doses of Individual Antioxidants on the Growth of Cancer and Normal Cells

Beta-Carotene and Vitamin A

Both beta-carotene and vitamin A (13-cis-retinoic acid and other analogs of retinoic acid) inhibit the growth of some cancer cells growing in culture as well as in vivo, without affecting the growth of most normal cells. They also convert some cancer cells to more normal-like cells. The extent of growth inhibition and differentiation depends on the type of tumor cells. Several reviews and articles have been published on this issue (Garewal 1995; Meyskens 1995; Prakash, Krinsky, and Russell 2000; Simeone and Tari 2005; Murakami et al. 2002). In a placebo-controlled trial, the effects of therapeutic doses of beta-carotene (180 mg per week) alone or in combination with vitamin A (100,000 IU per week) was evaluated on fishermen from Kerala, India, who chewed tobacco-containing betel quids and had well-developed oral leukopla-kia, a premalignant lesion. The capsules were given twice weekly for six months. The patients were allowed to continue chewing betel quids in their accustomed manner. The results showed that the beta-carotene supplementation produced complete remission in about 15 percent, and the combination of beta-carotene and vitamin A caused complete remis-sion in 27.5 percent of patients; in the placebo group, complete remis-sion was observed in only 3 percent (Stich et al. 1988). In addition, the development of new leukoplakia was strongly inhibited in groups taking both beta-carotene and vitamin A. A higher therapeutic dose of vitamin A alone (13-cis-retinoic acid at 200,000 IU per week) led to complete remission in 27 percent of patients with oral leukoplakia (Stich 1991).

Laboratory experiments have shown that carotenoids, including beta-carotene, alpha-carotene, lycopene, and canthaxanthin inhibit the growth of prostate-cancer cells and colon-cancer cells in culture (Okuno et al. 1998; Williams et al. 2000; Briviba et al. 2001; Hwang and Bowen 2004; van Breemen and Pajkovic 2008). Vitamin A (reti-noic acid) at therapeutic doses inhibits the growth of human cancer of the head and neck (Meyskens 1995). The recurrence of melanoma after surgical removal is high (30 to 75 percent), depending on the stage of the cancer. But reports show that the combination of BCG vaccine with vitamin A at a therapeutic dose (100,000 IU per day), taken for eighteen months, slightly increases the disease-free period in stage I and II melanoma compared with BCG vaccine alone (Meyskens 1982). The side effects of this treatment included dry skin and mild depression. The administration of BCG alone has produced varying degrees of tumor regression. One of the actions of BCG is increased immune function, which helps to inhibit the growth of melanoma cells.

A pronounced beneficial effect of 13-cis-retinoic acid at therapeutic doses on cutaneous T-cell lymphoma (mycosis fungoides) has been observed. In one study eight of twelve patients responded well, and four of twelve showed nearly complete cure (Meyskens 1995). Beneficial effects of therapeutic doses of vitamin A were also noted in some patients with epithelial tumors. Vitamin A alone was ineffective in treating non-epithelial cancer.

Although vitamin A and its analogs—retinoids—at high therapeutic doses alone or in combination with beta-carotene or BCG vaccine have produced beneficial effects in treating some tumors, they may not have optimal benefits. In addition, the toxicity of high therapeutic doses of vitamin A (100,000 to 200,000 IU) may be a limiting factor. However, laboratory data show that if vitamin A and beta-carotene are used together in multiple-micronutrient preparations containing other dietary antioxidants, the effective therapeutic dose may be lower. Individually, retinoids or beta-carotene at low preventive doses can actually increase the growth of certain cancer cells. For this and other reasons, the use of a single micronutrient at preventive doses in cancer treatment has no scientific basis.

Vitamin C

Although laboratory studies have shown that vitamin C reduces the growth and migration of several types of human cancer cells in laboratory studies without affecting the growth of normal cells (Lee et al. 2008; Wybieralska et al. 2008; Hong et al. 2007. Sun et al. 2006; Gonzalez et al. 2005; Prasad et al. 1979), its role in treating human cancer has become controversial. This may be in part because the doses of vitamin C used in the study have varied from preventive to therapeutic. The fact that vitamin C prevents the migration of cancer cells suggests that it may play a role in preventing the spread of tumors to other organs. Researchers Dr. Ewan Cameron, Nobel Prize winner

Dr. Linus Pauling, and Dr. Leibowitz (1979) have reported that oral administration of therapeutic doses of vitamin C (sodium ascorbate, 5 to 10 g per day) lengthens the survival time of patients with advanced cancer. These patients either were treated minimally with standard therapies or were not treated at all. Other scientists have reported that vitamin C administered orally at similar therapeutic doses was ineffective in improving the survival time of patients with terminal cancer (Creagan, Moerrtel, and O'Fallon 1979). These patients were treated extensively with radiation therapy and chemotherapy before vitamin C treatment was started. The exact reasons for the difference in results of these studies are not known but may be related to the different patient groups. An analysis of thirty-eight studies shows that treatment with high therapeutic doses of vitamin C or vitamin E alone produced some beneficial effects on survival of cancer patients.

It is interesting to note that in some alternative/complementary medicine practices, vitamin C in doses as high as 80 g are administered intravenously to patients with advanced disease who have failed all treatments. Claims have been made of the beneficial effect of this treatment on tumor regression, without toxicity. Therapeutic doses of vitamin C administered intravenously have been reported to kill some tumor cells but not normal cells. Both intraperitoneal and intravenous administration of therapeutic doses of vitamin C have been shown to decrease the growth of hepatoma (a liver cancer) in mice, whereas oral administration of the same dose was ineffective (Verrax and Calderon 2009). The intravenous route of injection is more effective in raising blood levels of vitamin C to therapeutic concentrations than intraperitoneal or oral administration in rats (Chen et al. 2007; Chen et al. 2005). These studies suggest that intravenous administration of therapeutic doses of vitamin C can produce some beneficial effects in cancer patients with poor prognosis and limited therapeutic options. In patients who have become unresponsive to all treatments, intravenous administration of therapeutic doses of vitamin C together with oral doses of a multiple micronutrient containing therapeutic doses of vitamin A, vitamin E (vitamin E acetate and vitamin E succinate), and beta-carotene may enhance efficacy.

One study has reported that local infusion of sodium ascorbate with copper and glycyl-glycyl-histidine, a peptide, caused complete regression of osteosarcoma (bone cancer) in one patient (Morishige 1983). This interesting study calls for further research. We should point out that the therapeutic doses of vitamin C alone may never be sufficient in the treatment of human cancer.

Vitamin C at preventive doses can increase the growth of some cancer cells, such as certain cancers of the salivary gland. Therefore, preventive doses of vitamin C alone should never be used in treating cancer.

Vitamin E

Vitamin E is sold commercially as alpha-tocopherol (a form present in the body and that is relatively unstable), alpha-tocopheryl acetate, alpha-tocopheryl nicotinate, and alpha-tocopheryl succinate, and in natural (d) or synthetic (dl) forms. The notion that all forms of vitamin E have only one function—namely, scavenging free radicals—and that they produce the same effects on cancer cells and normal cells is incorrect. In addition, when presented with both natural and synthetic forms, the body prefers the natural form of vitamin E and accumulates more of it than the synthetic form. In 1982 we discovered that alpha-tocopheryl succinate (vitamin E succinate) is the most effective form of vitamin E. It induces differentiation, inhibits growth, and promotes cell death in melanoma cells of mice (Prasad and Edwards-Prasad 1982). Therapeutic doses and a treatment time of three days or more were necessary to produce these effects. Other forms of vitamin E, such as alpha-tocopherol (vitamin E), alpha-tocopheryl acetate (vitamin E acetate), and alpha-tocopheryl nicotinate (vitamin E nicotinate) at the same therapeutic doses were ineffective. Since then more than two hundred studies on the effects of vitamin E succinate on the growth of several types of cancer and normal cells in culture and in tumor-bearing animal models have been published (Prasad et al. 2003). The results of these studies have shown that vitamin E succinate selectively inhibits the growth of cancer cells without affecting the growth of normal cells. Vitamin E succinate also inhibits the expression of androgen (male sex hormones) receptors in prostate-cancer cells but not in normal prostate epithelial cells in culture. (Increased expression of androgen receptors promotes growth of prostate-cancer cells.) Vitamin E succinate also reduces the levels of prostate-specific antigen, one of the commonly used markers of prostate-cancer progression and increased disease survival. Laboratory experiments have shown that the treatment of hormone-resistant human breast-cancer cells with vitamin E succinate makes them sensitive to standard therapy. These observations on the effect of vitamin E succinate on hormone-sensitive tumors, if true in humans, could have an enormous impact on improving the treatment of hormone-resistant tumors, such as breast cancer and prostate cancer.

Vitamin E succinate is degraded by the enzyme esterase, which may reduce its anticancer activity. Recently, several esterase-resistant analogs of vitamin E have been made in the laboratory. These include alpha-tocopheryl hemisuccinate, alpha-tocopheryl meleamide, alpha-tocopheryl malonate, alpha-tocopheryl oxalate, alpha-topopheryl oxbutyl sufonic acid, and alpha-tocopheryl oxyacetic acid. Some of these esterase-resistant analogs are toxic to both normal and cancer cells in culture, but they have not shown any toxicity in tumor-bearing animal models. Most studies with vitamin E have primarily utilized the intraperitoneal route of administration; however, some esterase-resistant vitamin E analogs maintained their effectiveness when administered orally. The toxicity of these analogs in humans remains uncertain. In addition, these analogs of vitamin E will require FDA approval for human use. Until then, therapeutic doses of vitamin E succinate, which has been consumed by humans for decades, is the best option as part of a multiple-micronutrient preparation for treating cancer. The references for this section have been included in a review (Prasad 2011).

Selenium

The references for this section have been included in a review (Prasad 2011). Laboratory studies have shown that therapeutic doses of selenium compounds (sodium selenite or seleno-L-methionine) inhibited the growth of several human and animal cancer cells, including breast cancer and prostate cancer, without affecting the growth of normal cells. Methyselenic, a selenium product formed in the body, is more effective than sodium selenite or seleno-L-methionine. The mechanisms of action of therapeutic doses of selenium on tumor growth appear to very complex and involve alterations in gene expression and the cell-signaling system. In addition, laboratory data also suggest that selenium treatment at therapeutic doses, like vitamin E treatment, markedly reduces androgen-receptor-mediated gene expression, including prostate-specific antigen, in human prostate-cancer cells. Increased levels of estrogen receptors on breast-tumor cells promote their growth. Selenium treatment reduces estrogen-receptor-alpha (ERalpha) expression in breast-tumor cells. Thus, selenium could be useful in the treatment of hormone-sensitive prostate cancer and breast cancer.

Laboratory studies have also shown that selenium together with genistein (one of the isoflavones found in fruits and vegetables) is more effective at killing cancer cells than the individual agents. Treatment of esophageal-cancer cells with sodium selenite plus zinc causes much more killing of cancer cells compared with the individual agent alone. Vitamin E succinate in combination with methyselenic acid is more effective in reducing the growth of prostate-cancer cells growing in petri dishes than either of these agents alone, without affecting the growth of normal prostate epithelial cells.

Treatment of tamoxifen-sensitive breast-cancer cells with methyselenic acid enhances the growth-inhibiting effects of tamoxifen; however, in tamoxifen-resistant breast-cancer cells, treatment with both methyselenic acid and tamoxifen limit the growth of cancer cells more than methyselenic acid alone.

Mixture of Dietary Antioxidants
The references for the subsequent sections have been included in a review (Prasad 2011).

Most clinical studies with antioxidants have utilized a single antioxidant, and this may be the cause of the inconsistent results. Our bodies have multiple antioxidants; using a single antioxidant for reducing the risk of human diseases makes no scientific sense. Furthermore, our laboratory research shows that a mixture of dietary antioxidants is more effective at killing cancer cells than are individual antioxidants. For example, carotenoids, retinoic acid (13-cis-retinoic acid), vitamin C (calcium ascorbate), and vitamin E succinate at low therapeutic doses did not inhibit the growth of human melanoma cells in culture. However, the mixture of these antioxidants at the same doses reduced the growth of cancer cells by about 50 percent (see Table 8.1). However, when a dose of vitamin C that inhibited the growth of cancer cells by about 35 percent was added to the mixture, it reduced the growth by about 87 percent. These results suggest that a mixture of antioxidants should be used in any clinical studies that investigate the effectiveness of antioxidants in reducing the growth of tumor cells in humans.

TABLE 8.1. EFFECT OF A MIXTURE OF FOUR ANTIOXIDANTS ON THE GROWTH OF HUMAN MELANOMA CELLS IN CULTURE

Treatments	Cell Number (percent of controls)
Vit C (50 µg/ml)	102 ± 5[a]
PC (10 µg/ml)	96 ± 2
Alpha-TS (10 µg/ml)	102 ± 3
RA (7.5 µg/ml)	103 ± 3
Vit C (50 µg/ml) + PC (10 µg/ml) + alpha-TS (10 µg/ml) + RA (7.5 µg/ml)	56 ± 3
Vit C (100 µg/ml)	64 ± 3
Vit C (100 µg/ml) + PC (10 µg/ml) + alpha-TS (10 µg/ml) + RA (7.5 µg/ml)	13 ± 1

µg = micrograms PC = carotenoids originally referred to as beta-carotene. This is a more soluble fraction of carotenoids without the presence of beta-carotene.	a = standard error of the mean Vit C = sodium ascorbate alpha-TS = alpha-tocopheryl succinate RA = 13-cis-retinoic acid

From: K. N. Prasad, *Micronutrients in Health and Disease*, Boca Raton, Fla.: Francis and Taylor Publishing Groups, 2011.

Combination of vitamins A, C, and E (vitamin E succinate) and carotenoids reduced the growth of cancer cells by about 87 percent, whereas these antioxidants individually have no effect on the growth of cancer cells.

Vitamin D

Laboratory experiments show that 1-alpha-hydroxyvitamin D_3 reduces the growth of cells of certain tumors, for example, melanoma, hepatocellular carcinoma (a liver cancer), and myeloid leukemia (a kind of blood cancer). It also converts some cancer cells, such as human leukemia cells, to more normal-like cells. Vitamin D is fairly nontoxic at therapeutic doses, at least for a short period of time. Laboratory or clinical studies of the effect of vitamin D in combination with antioxidants on tumor cells and normal cells have not been performed.

N-acetylcysteine (NAC) and Alpha-lipoic Acid

The role of endogenous antioxidants on the growth of cancer or normal cells has not been adequately studied. Several laboratory studies show that N-acetylcysteine (NAC), a glutathione-elevating agent, at therapeutic doses reduced the growth of several animal and human cancer cells. NAC treatment also reduced the incidence and number of lymphoma tumors in mice carrying a mutated gene (Atm) and increased their life span. NAC at therapeutic doses can reportedly act as an anti-angiogenesis agent that causes vascular collapse in the tumor, thereby inhibiting its growth. Laboratory studies suggest that alpha-lipoic acid (a glutathione-elevating agent that also acts as an antioxidant in its own right) at therapeutic doses kills cancer cells without killing normal cells.

Coenzyme Q10

There are no significant data on the effects of coenzyme Q10 alone on growth or survival of tumor cells in laboratory experiments.

Antioxidant Enzymes

Superoxide dismutase (SOD) is an antioxidant enzyme that protects cells from free-radical damage. It requires manganese (Mn) for its activity and is located in the mitochondria of the cell. Laboratory studies show that if the activity of Mn-SOD is increased in cancer cells, the growth of those cells is decreased. This phenomenon has been demonstrated in melanoma cells and glioma cells. The relevance of this observation in treating human cancer is not certain, because it is difficult to enhance the activity of Mn-SOD in tumors growing in the body.

Vitamin B₆

Some animal studies have reported that supplementation with vitamin B_6, one of the B-complex vitamins, at therapeutic doses enhances the growth of human breast-cancer cells transplanted into athymic mice (mice with no thymus gland that cannot reject cancer cells from other species). However, another study reports that restriction of vitamin B_6 reduces the growth of breast-cancer cells growing in petri dishes. The role of vitamin B_6 in cancer growth remains uncertain at this time. Nevertheless, supplementation with high doses of vitamin B_6 (50 mg or more per day) should be avoided. However, lower doses of vitamin B_6 (less than 10 mg per day) are needed, because radiation therapy and chemotherapy decrease the levels of micronutrients, including vitamin B_6.

Treatment Schedules

Laboratory studies show that treatment time with therapeutic doses of antioxidants is also very important in order to produce a differential effect on normal and cancer cells. A short exposure time of a few hours may not cause significant killing and/or growth inhibition of cancer cells. At least twenty-four hours or more are needed to observe a significant reduction in growth and/or killing of cancer cells without affecting the growth of normal cells.

EFFECTS OF THERAPEUTIC DOSES OF INDIVIDUAL ANTIOXIDANTS ON GENE-EXPRESSION PROFILES IN CANCER CELLS

Several laboratory studies have reported that therapeutic doses of antioxidants or their derivatives inhibit the growth of cancer cells but not of normal cells. The studies on the expression of genes that are involved in differentiation (converting cancer cells to normal-like cells), growth inhibition, and apoptosis (a form of cell death) reveal that retinoids, vitamin E (vitamin E succinate and vitamin E), and beta-carotene inhibit as well as stimulate the levels of some cell-signaling systems and gene expression, which can lead to a decreased cell-proliferation rate and increased differentiation and/or apoptosis. Some of the changes in gene-expression profiles following treatment with therapeutic doses of individual antioxidants include inhibitory and stimulatory events. Inhibitory events include decreased expression of c-myc, H-ras N-myc, mutated p53, the activity of protein kinase C, caspase, tumor necrosis factor, transcriptional factor E2F, and Fas. Stimulatory events include increased expression of wild type p53, p21, transforming growth factor beta (TGF-beta), and the connexin gene. Marked changes in gene expression have been observed as early as thirty minutes after treatment of neuroblastoma cells with a therapeutic dose of vitamin E succinate. The above changes in gene expression may be one of the major factors that account for the growth-inhibiting effect of vitamin E succinate on cancer cells.

Vitamin E succinate also reduces the expression of vascular endothelial growth factor (VEGF) and thus acts as an anti-angiogenesis factor at a therapeutic dose that is not toxic to normal cells. This observation is very exciting, because the toxicity of available anti-angiogenesis drugs limits their usefulness in treating human cancers.

EFFECTS OF PREVENTIVE DOSES
OF INDIVIDUAL ANTIOXIDANTS ON
GROWTH OF CANCER CELLS

The effects of preventive doses of antioxidants on cancer and normal cells are different from those produced by therapeutic doses. Several laboratory studies have reported that preventive doses of antioxidants can increase the growth of cancer cells. For example, our research has shown that preventive doses of vitamin C can stimulate the growth of parotid-gland cancer. Preventive doses of retinol and beta-carotene also increase the growth of pulmonary adenocarcinoma (a form of lung cancer). Laboratory studies have reported that retinoic acid at preventive doses enhances the proliferation of human squamous-cell carcinoma. Preventive doses of selenomethionine have also been reported to increase the growth of some cancer cells in culture. Thus, we recommend therapeutic doses of multiple antioxidants for cancer treatment, in consultation with the patient's doctor.

STUDIES ON THE EFFECTS OF
THERAPEUTIC DOSES OF INDIVIDUAL
ANTIOXIDANTS IN COMBINATION
WITH STANDARD OR EXPERIMENTAL THERAPY
ON GROWTH OF CANCER AND NORMAL CELLS

As previously mentioned, oncologists often discourage cancer patients from taking antioxidants during radiation therapy, chemotherapy, or experimental therapy because of concerns that antioxidants may protect cancer cells from free-radical damage.

Several laboratory and a few clinical studies suggest that this fear may not be justified. Some of these studies are described here.

EFFECTS OF THERAPEUTIC DOSES OF INDIVIDUAL ANTIOXIDANTS ON RADIATION- AND CHEMOTHERAPEUTIC AGENT–INDUCED DAMAGE IN CANCER CELLS AND NORMAL CELLS

Results of laboratory experiments indicate that therapeutic doses of beta-carotene and vitamins A, C, and E can intensify the growth-inhibiting effects of standard therapeutic agents (radiation and certain chemotherapeutic drugs) and experimental therapeutic agents (heat, sodium butyrate, and some interferons) on cancer cells without affecting the growth of normal cells. The extent of enhancement depends on the types of tumor cells, the types of micronutrients, and the types of cancer-therapeutic agents. The enhancement of the effects of such treatments by micronutrients is discussed in the following sections.

ENHANCEMENT OF THE BENEFICIAL EFFECTS OF X-IRRADIATION WITH THERAPEUTIC DOSES OF VITAMIN A AND BETA-CAROTENE

Laboratory studies suggest that vitamin A or beta-carotene alone at therapeutic doses inhibit the growth of breast-cancer cells. Vitamin A (retinyl palmitate) together with radiation, or beta-carotene with radiation, produced a cure rate of more than 90 percent in mice (Seifter, Padawar, and Levenson 1984) (see Table 8.2). Cancers were completely cured in mice given both vitamin A and radiation. This treatment with a micronutrient reduced the toxicity of radiation on normal cells. Retinoids enhance the cytotoxicity of cisplatin on human ovarian cancer cells transplanted into athymic mice. Retinoic acid heightened the cell-killing effect of radiation on cancer cells by inhibiting the repair process more effectively in cancer cells compared to normal cells. Retinoic acid in combination with interferon-alpha-2a enhanced radiation-induced damage on cancer of head and neck (squamous cell carcinoma) in humans.

TABLE 8.2. EFFECT OF VITAMIN A, BETA-CAROTENE, AND LOCAL X-IRRADIATION ON SURVIVAL OF MICE WITH TRANSPLANTED BREAST ADENOCARCINOMA

Treatments	Number of Mice	One-Year Survival
Control	24	0
3,000 rads, single dose	24	0
Vitamin A	24	0
Beta-carotene	24	0
Vitamin A plus X-ray	24	22
Beta-Carotene plus X-ray	24	22

Diets were supplemented with vitamin A (3,000 IU per mouse) and beta-carotene (270 mcg per mouse), and these doses were about ten times greater than the RDA for mice.

From K. N. Prasad, *Micronutrients in Health and Disease,* Boca Raton, Fla.: Francis and Taylor Publishing Groups, 2011.

A clinical study has shown that retinoic acid and interferon alpha2a enhanced the effectiveness of radiation therapy on locally advanced cervical cancer (Lippman et al. 1992). Another human study revealed that therapeutic doses (100 mg per day) of beta-carotene reduced radiation-induced mucositis (damage to mucous membranes of the mouth) without interfering with the efficacy of radiation therapy in patients with cancer of the head and neck (Mills 1988). These human studies are important because they show the potential value of antioxidants in improving the current management of human cancer.

In spite of any beneficial results obtained by combining therapeutic doses of vitamin A or beta-carotene, this strategy is not optimal. Best results may be obtained by using a multiple micronutrient containing therapeutic doses of vitamin A and beta-carotene. Because of the toxicity of therapeutic doses of retinoids in humans, we do not recommend adding this analog of vitamin A in any multiple-vitamin preparation for therapeutic purposes.

ENHANCEMENT OF THE BENEFICIAL EFFECTS OF X-IRRADIATION WITH THERAPEUTIC DOSES OF VITAMIN C

Therapeutic doses of vitamin C increase the growth-inhibiting effects of X-irradiation on neuroblastoma cells but have failed to enhance the effect of irradiation on glioma cells (a form of brain cancer). Vitamin C protects the ovary cells in hamsters against radiation damage. Vitamin C in combination with X-irradiation lengthens the survival time of mice with tumor cells growing in the fluid of the abdominal cavity more than irradiation alone. Therapeutic doses of dehydroascorbic acid (DA), the major degradation product of vitamin C, increase the cell-killing effect of X-irradiation on hypoxic (less-oxygenated) tumor cells, which are normally very resistant to radiation therapy. No human studies with vitamin C alone in combination with radiation therapy have been performed.

ENHANCEMENT OF THE BENEFICIAL EFFECTS OF X-IRRADIATION WITH THERAPEUTIC DOSES OF VITAMIN E AND SELENIUM

Vitamin E

Laboratory experiments have shown that therapeutic doses of vitamin E (vitamin E succinate and the aqueous form of vitamin E acetate) increase the damaging effects of X-irradiation on neuroblastoma, glioma, cervical-cancer, and ovarian-cancer cells, whereas preventive doses of vitamin E are ineffective. Vitamin E succinate at therapeutic doses enhances the levels of radiation-induced chromosomal (genetic) damage in several human cancer cells but protects normal cells (fibroblasts). This form of vitamin E also increases the growth-inhibiting effect of gamma-radiation on human breast-cancer cells and human cervical-cancer in culture.

In a clinical study ninety-one patients with lung cancer were divided into two groups. Forty-four patients received an oral dose of pentoxifylline (400 mg three times a day) and vitamin E (300 mg twice a day) during the entire period of radiation therapy, while the other forty-seven patients received only radiation therapy. The first group also received 400 mg of pentoxifylline and 300 mg of vitamin E once a day for a period of three months after completion of radiation therapy. The median follow-up period was thirteen months. The results showed that radiation-induced lung toxicity was reduced in the vitamin E–treated group compared with the nontreated group (Misirlioglu et al. 2007).

Selenium

Seleno-L-methionine, a common form of selenium used in multiple-micronutrient preparations, at therapeutic doses enhances the cell-killing effect of ionizing radiation on two lung-cancer cell lines but does not have the same effect on normal lung fibroblasts in culture. This selective effect of selenium on tumor-cell response to radiation is similar to those produced by other antioxidants.

ENHANCEMENT OF THE BENEFICIAL EFFECTS OF CHEMOTHERAPEUTIC AGENTS WITH THERAPEUTIC DOSES OF VITAMIN A AND BETA-CAROTENE

Laboratory studies have shown that vitamin A (retinyl palmitate) or synthetic beta-carotene at therapeutic doses (tenfold higher than RDA values) together with cyclophosphamide, a commonly used chemotherapeutic agent, or beta-carotene with this chemotherapeutic agent produced a cure rate of more than 90 percent in animals with transplanted breast cancer (see Table 10). This micronutrient treatment also reduced the toxicity of chemotherapeutic agents on normal cells.

The synthetic retinoid fenretinide has reduced the growth of human ovarian cancer transplanted in athymic mice and increased the antitumor activity of cisplatin. Retinoic acid in combination with tamoxifen inhibits the growth of human melanoma cells more than the individual agents alone.

Beta-carotene and lycopene at therapeutic doses also enhance the growth-inhibiting effect of docetaxel on human estrogen-positive breast cancer cells in culture. No studies have been performed to evaluate the role of beta-carotene or vitamin A in combination with chemotherapy in humans.

ENHANCEMENT OF THE BENEFICIAL EFFECTS OF CHEMOTHERAPEUTIC AGENTS WITH THERAPEUTIC DOSES OF VITAMIN C

Therapeutic doses of vitamin C increase the effect of several other chemotherapeutic agents, such as 5-fluorouracil (5-FU), Adriamycin (also known as doxorubicin), bleomycin, and vincristine, on neuroblastoma cells in culture. Vitamin C at therapeutic doses increases the antitumor activity of doxorubicin, cisplatin, and paclitaxel in human breast cancer cells in culture. It also enhances the growth-inhibiting effect of 5-FU and cisplatin on esophageal-cancer cells in culture.

Therapeutic dose of vitamin C (sodium ascorbate) in combination with CCNU (a commonly used chemotherapeutic agent) are reported to enhance the survival rate of mice with leukemia by two, compared with CCNU alone. No studies have been performed to evaluate the role of vitamin C in combination with chemotherapy in humans.

ENHANCEMENT OF THE BENEFICIAL EFFECTS OF CHEMOTHERAPEUTIC AGENTS WITH THERAPEUTIC DOSES OF VITAMIN E AND SELENIUM

Vitamin E

Vitamin E succinate at therapeutic doses amplifies the effect of many chemotherapeutic agents on several tumor cells in cell culture and in animals. Vitamin E succinate enhances the cell-killing effect of Adriamycin on human prostate-cancer cells in culture and at therapeutic doses increases the growth-inhibiting effect of Adriamycin on human cervical cancer cells in culture, but it does not produce this effect on normal human cells (Table 8.3). Vitamin E succinate also enhances the effect of carmustine (a commonly used drug for brain tumors) on rat glioma cells in culture. One study has reported that the aqueous form of vitamin E was more effective in limiting the growth of human colon-cancer cells growing in athymic mice than 5-fluorouracil (5-FU) alone. The combination of vitamin E and 5-FU was much more potent than the individual agents in reducing tumor growth. An aqueous form of vitamin E, alpha-tocopheryl acetate, at therapeutic doses enhanced the growth-inhibiting effect of vincristine on neuroblastoma cells in culture. Vitamin E (alpha-tocopherol) protected against cisplatin-induced toxicity without interfering with its antitumor activity in human melanoma cells transplanted in athymic mice. These studies emphasize that the appropriate form of vitamin E must be used in any clinical trial for the treatment of cancer. As mentioned previously, we advise using therapeutic doses of multiple rather than single micronutrients in combination with standard cancer therapy.

TABLE 8.3. MODIFICATION OF ADRIAMYCIN EFFECT BY VITAMIN E SUCCINATE ON HUMAN CERVICAL-CANCER CELLS (HELA) AND HUMAN NORMAL SKIN FIBROBLASTS IN CULTURE

Treatment	HeLa Cells	Normal fibroblasts
Solvent Control	99 ± 2.6	104 ± 3.4
Adriamycin (0.1 µg/ml)	57 ± 6.2	77 ± 2.4
Vitamin E succinate (10 µg/ml)	99 ± 1.6	101 ± 3.7
Adriamycin (0.1 µg/ml) plus vitamin E succinate	20 ± 7.9	77 ± 1.7
Adriamycin (0.25 µg/ml)	14 ± 2.9	68 ± 1.0
Adriamycin (0.25 µg/ml)plus vitamin E succinate	5 ± 0.8	62 ± 1.8

µg = micrograms

Growth of cells in experimental groups was expressed as a percent of the untreated control group and expressed as an average (mean) value ± SEM (standard error of the mean).

Vitamin E succinate treatment enhanced the growth-inhibiting effect of Adriamycin on cancer cells (HeLa cells derived from human carcinoma of cervix) but not on human normal cells (fibroblasts).

From K. N. Prasad, *Micronutrients in Health and Disease,* Boca Raton, Fla.: Francis and Taylor Publishing Groups, 2011.

Peripheral neuropathy (numbness of the extremities) is one of the serious side effects of certain types of chemotherapeutic agents, such as cisplatin. Supplementation with a therapeutic dose (600 or 300 mg per day orally) of vitamin E reduced cisplatin-induced peripheral neuropathy from about 69 percent to 21 percent (Argyriou et al. 2006; Argyriou et al. 2005; Pace et al. 2003). Supplementation with therapeutic doses of vitamin E also improved immune function in patients with advanced colon and rectal cancer (Malmberg et al. 2002). These studies reveal the usefulness of vitamin E in cancer treatment. Therefore, we recommend adding therapeutic doses of vitamin E to a multiple-micronutrient preparation for optimal benefit.

Selenium

Therapeutic doses of selenium compounds (sodium selenite and selenosulfate) decrease cisplatin-induced toxicity without compromising its efficacy on the growth of tumor cells in animal models. However, selenosulfate appeared to be less toxic than sodium selenite. In certain animal tumors the combination of selenosulfate and cisplatin reportedly produced a cure rate of 87.5 percent, compared with a 25-percent cure rate in the cisplatin-treated group.

Treatment with therapeutic doses of sodium selenite and selenous acid decreases the growth of cancer cells that are resistant to 5-FU, a commonly used chemotherapeutic agent. Supplementation with selenium enhances the growth-inhibiting effects of taxol and Adriamycin (doxorubicin) on several tumor cell lines in culture. Diphenylmethyl selenocyanate, another selenium compound, improved the antitumor activity of cyclophosphamide and at the same time reduced its toxicity. Thus, there are a substantial number of laboratory studies showing that selenium compounds at therapeutic doses increase the antitumor activity of several types of chemotherapeutic agents on cancer cells, while protecting or having no effect on normal cells. Organic selenium at a therapeutic dose (0.2 mg per day in mice or 10 mg per kg of body weight per day) enhanced the treatment efficacy of some chemotherapeutic agents in athymic mice with tumors derived from human squamous-cell carcinoma of the head and neck. Similar observations in human cancer would be very exciting.

A review of several clinical studies revealed that supplementation with selenium in combination with radiation therapy or chemotherapy did not provide any beneficial effects in reducing the toxicity of therapy or improving the quality of life of cancer patients (Dennert and Horneber 2006). Preventive doses of selenium were used in these studies; therefore, the above results were not unexpected. Although the use of a single antioxidant increases the effectiveness of radiation or chemotherapeutic agents on cancer cells in the laboratory experiments, it has frequently produced inconsistent results in humans. Therefore, we do not recommend using a single antioxidant for cancer treatment.

ENHANCEMENT OF THE BENEFICIAL EFFECTS OF CHEMOTHERAPEUTIC AGENTS WITH THERAPEUTIC DOSES OF GLUTATHIONE-ELEVATING AGENTS (N-ACETYLCYSTEINE AND ALPHA-LIPOIC ACID)

Intraperitoneal administration of N-acetylcysteine (NAC) at a high therapeutic dose (200 mg per kg of body weight) enhances the growth-inhibiting effect of 5-FU on human colon cancer cells growing in athymic mice without increasing the toxicity on normal cells.

Intravenous injection of NAC (800 mg per kg of body weight) has been effective in reducing cisplatin-induced toxicity on nerve cells in normal rats, whereas the intraperitoneal route was ineffective. In another animal study, intravenous administration of NAC (400 mg per kg of body weight) was effective in reducing cisplatin-induced damage to the kidney, whereas intraperitoneal injection was ineffective. One study has reported that intraperitoneal injection of NAC at a high therapeutic dose of 1 g per kg of body weight in combination with the chemotherapeutic agent doxorubicin reduced tumor size and metastases in mice with transplanted melanoma tumor cells.

As mentioned earlier, sensory neuropathy (damage to sensory nerves) is a serious side effect of certain chemotherapeutic agents. In a clinical study, oral supplementation with a high therapeutic dose of 1,200 mg NAC in combination with standard chemotherapy (oxaliplatin, 5-FU, and leucovorin) markedly reduced the incidence of sensory neuropathy from 57 percent to 7 percent in colon-cancer patients with metastases (Lin et al. 2006). In another clinical study, intravenous infusion of 1,500 mg/m2 of glutathione fifteen minutes before administration of oxaliplatin markedly reduced sensory neuropathy from 42 percent to 14 percent (Cascinu 2002). It is important to point out that treatment with endogenous antioxidants (glutathione or the glutathione-elevating agent NAC) did not decrease the antitumor activity of oxaliplatin.

Patients with advanced terminal pancreatic cancer often lose hope for any chance of prolonged survival with a good-quality life. Intravenous administration of therapeutic doses of alpha-lipoic acid together with a low-dose naltrexone (a chemotherapeutic agent) and a healthy lifestyle program greatly improve survival time and quality of life in some of these patients (Berkson, Rubin, and Berkson, 2006). High therapeutic doses of glutathione-elevating agents may be needed to reduce the toxicity of chemotherapy.

ENHANCEMENT OF THE BENEFICIAL EFFECTS OF CHEMOTHERAPEUTIC AGENTS WITH THERAPEUTIC DOSES OF COENZYME Q10

In a clinical study, oral supplementation with a therapeutic dose (390 mg per day) of coenzyme Q10 in combination with standard therapy markedly reduced the size of breast cancer and metastases in humans (Lockwood et al. 1994, 1995). A review of six studies revealed that oral administration of coenzyme Q10 in combination with anthracyclines reduced cardiac and liver toxicity (Roffe, Schmidt, and Ernst 2004). Oral administration of coenzyme Q10 (400 mg per day) in combination with low-dose interferon-alpha-2b for a period of three years decreased the rates of tumor recurrence in patients with stage I and stage II melanoma after surgical removal (Rusciani 2007).

Tamoxifen has been found to increase disease-free states and overall survival in women after primary surgery for breast cancer. However, this drug increases levels of triglycerides and induces angiogenesis (formation of new blood vessels that can theoretically increase the risk of metastasis). Oral supplementation of a preventive dose of coenzyme Q10 (100 mg per day) and low-dose tamoxifen reduces the levels of triglycerides and angiogenesis (Sachdanandam 2008). In one study a mixture of micronutrients containing 100 mg coenzyme Q10, 50 mg niacin, and 10 mg riboflavin, when administered orally in combination with tamoxifen daily for ninety days, reduced the levels of triglycerides to near normal and decreased angiogenesis in patients with breast cancer (Yuvaraj et al. 2007). In a randomized clinical trial involving eighty-four breast-cancer patiensts, the same preparation of micronutrients, in combination with tamoxifen, when administered orally for a period of forty-five and ninety days, decreased the levels of pro-angiogenic factors and increased the levels of anti-angiogenic factors (Premkumar 2008). These observations are important, because pro-angiogenesis factors promote spread of tumors to other organs, whereas anti-angiogenesis factors prevent it. Thus, therapeutic doses of coenzyme Q10 may be very useful in reducing the toxicity of chemotherapy.

ENHANCEMENT OF THE BENEFICIAL EFFECTS OF CHEMOTHERAPEUTIC AGENTS WITH THERAPEUTIC DOSES OF A MIXTURE OF ANTIOXIDANTS

We have reported that a mixture of antioxidants containing therapeutic doses of retinoic acid, vitamin C, vitamin E succinate, and carotenoids in combination with DTIC [5-(3,3-dimethyl-l-triazeno)-imidazole-4-carboxamide, also called decarbazine], tamoxifen, cisplatin, or interferon-alpha-2a limits the growth of human melanoma cells more than that produced by the individual agents (see Table 8.4). Another study has reported that a mixture of dietary antioxidants (vitamin C, 100 mg; alpha-tocopherol, 10 mcg; and beta-carotene, 10 mcg per milliliter) by itself increased cell killing from 4 percent to 15 percent, whereas carboplatin and paclitaxel increased it to 22 percent and 87 percent, respectively. However, the mixture of dietary antioxidants enhanced the cell-killing effect of paclitaxel and carboplatin. The most pronounced effect was observed when the antioxidant mixture was given before treatment with chemotherapeutic agents, followed by paclitaxel treatment for twenty-four hours and then followed by carboplatin treatment for twenty-four hours. This suggests that multiple antioxidants are also effective in enhancing the effect of certain chemotherapeutic agents on cancer cells.

TABLE 8.4. ENHANCEMENT OF THE EFFECT OF CERTAIN CHEMOTHERAPEUTIC AGENTS BY A MIXTURE OF FOUR ANTIOXIDANTS ON HUMAN MELANOMA CELLS IN CULTURE

Treatments	Cell Number (Percent of Controls)
Solvent	101 ± 4[a]
Cisplatin (1 µg/ml)	67 ± 4
Treatments	Cell Number (Percent of Controls)
Antioxidant mixture	56 ± 3
Cisplatin + antioxidant mixture	38 ± 2
Tamoxifen (2 µg/ml)	81 ± 3
Tamoxifen + antioxidant mixture	30 ± 2
DTIC (100 µg/ml)	71 ± 2
DTIC + antioxidant mixture	38 ± 2
Interferon- alpha2b	82 ± 5
Interferon- alpha2b + antioxidant mixture	29 ± 1

a = average (mean value) + standard error of the mean
Polar carotenoids were originally referred to as beta-carotene
Vitamin C, 50 µg/ml; polar carotenoids, 10 µg/ml; alpha-tocopheryl succinate, 10 µg/ml and 13-cis-retinoic acid, 7.5 µg/ml were added simultaneously
µg = micrograms

Antioxidant mixture enhanced the growth-inhibiting effect of certain chemotherapeutic agents on cancer cells.

From K. N. Prasad, *Micronutrients in Health and Disease,* Boca Raton, Fla.: Francis and Taylor Publishing Groups, 2011.

One study evaluated the effect of a multiple-micronutrient preparation in combination with standard therapy in thirty-two patients with advanced breast cancer, aged thirty-two to eighty-one years. The micronutrient preparation contained 2,850 mg vitamin C, 2,500 IU vitamin E, 32.5 IU beta-carotene, 387 mcg selenium, secondary vitamins and minerals, essential fatty acids (1.2 g gamma-linolenic acid and 3.5 g omega-3 fatty acids), and 90 mg coenzyme Q10 and was administered orally. None of the patients died during the study period (the expected number was four), there was no evidence of further metastasis, and there was improved quality of life (no weight loss, and reduced use of pain medications). In addition, six patients showed apparent partial remission.

Eighteen non-randomized patients with small-cell lung cancer received multiple-antioxidant treatment in combination with chemotherapy and/or radiation. The median survival time was markedly enhanced, and patients tolerated chemotherapy and radiation well (Jaakkola et al. 1992). Similar observations were made in several private-practice settings (Lamson and Brignall 1999). A randomized pilot trial has been completed with high-dose multiple micronutrients including dietary antioxidants and their derivatives (Sevak, a multiple-vitamin preparation, 8 grams vitamin C as calcium ascorbate, 800 IU vitamin E as vitamin E succinate, and 60 mg natural beta-carotene) divided into two oral doses, one in the morning and one in the evening, for patients with up to stage III breast cancer and receiving radiation therapy (Walker et al. 2002). Twenty-five patients were in the radiation group and twenty-two patients were in the group receiving radiation therapy and antioxidants. In the follow-up period of twenty-two months, during which no maintenance micronutrient supplements were given, one patient in the radiation group developed a new cancer in the opposite breast, and another in the same group developed LCIS (lobular carcinoma in situ) in the opposite breast. In the combination group, no new tumors developed.

A randomized trial with high-dose multiple antioxidants and involving 136 patients with stage IIIb and stage IV non-small-cell lung cancer was conducted to evaluate the efficacy of an antioxidant preparation in modifying the response of tumor cells to chemotherapy (paclitaxel and carboplatin). The control group received only chemotherapy, whereas the treatment group received chemotherapy plus high-dose multiple antioxidants (6,100 mg vitamin C as ascorbic acid, 1,050 mg vitamin E as dl-alpha-tocopheryl succinate, 60 mg synthetic beta-carotene). The preparation also contained selenium, copper sulfate, and zinc sulfate. Antioxidants were administered once a day orally and continued for the entire treatment period. The follow-up period was two years. The results showed that 48.6 percent of patients in the control group (seventy-two patients) completed six cycles of chemotherapy, whereas in the treatment group (sixty-four patients) 56.2 percent completed six cycles of chemotherapy. In the control group there was no complete response (CR); however, two patients in the treatment group had a complete response. The overall survival in the control group at one and two years was 32.9 percent and 11.1 percent, respectively, whereas it was 39.1 and 15.6 percent, respectively, in the treatment group (See Table 8.5). The mean survival time in the control and treatment groups was nine months and eleven months, respectively (Pathak et al. 2005). There was no difference in toxicity between the two groups. The sample size was small and there was no significant difference on any measures of outcome. Nevertheless, these results do not support the concern of oncologists that high doses of multiple antioxidants may protect cancer cells from the free-radical damage induced by radiation therapy or chemotherapy.

TABLE 8.5. PRELIMINARY RESULTS OF A RANDOMIZED CLINICAL TRIAL USING HIGH-DOSE MULTIPLE ANTIOXIDANTS IN COMBINATION WITH CHEMOTHERAPY

Tumor response and Survival	Chemotherapy Arm (Number of Patients = 72)	Chemo + Antioxidant (Number of Patients = 64)
Complete response	0	2
Partial response	32 percent	45 percent
Overall survival at 1 year	2.9 percent	39.1 percent
Overall survival at 2 years	11.1 percent	15.6 percent
Median survival time	9 months	11 months

Antioxidant mixture contained ascorbic acid, 6,100 mg; dl-alpha-tocopheryl succinate, 1,050 mg; beta-carotene (synthetic), 60 mg. The preparation also contained copper sulfate, manganese sulfate, zinc sulfate, and selenium. Antioxidant was administered daily orally forty-eight hours before chemotherapy and continued every day for the entire treatment period.

From K. N. Prasad, *Micronutrients in Health and Disease*, Boca Raton, Fla.: Francis and Taylor Publishing Groups, 2011.

Based on the beneficial effects of multiple antioxidants in combination with standard therapy on two patients with ovarian cancer (Drisko, Chapman, and Hunter, 2003), Dr. Jeanne Drisko has started a new trial with multiple antioxidants on ovarian-cancer patients. Cell-culture studies, animal studies, and limited human studies suggest that a well-designed trial with therapeutic doses of multiple antioxidants administered orally before and during the entire treatment period is urgently needed.

Combination of Vitamin C or Vitamin E with Other Therapeutic Agents

In a study, alpha-tocopheryl succinate (vitamin E succinate) in combination with tumor necrosis factor–related apoptosis-inducing ligand (TRAIL), a potential chemotherapeutic agent, and dendritic cells (which increase immune function) caused complete tumor regression without causing adverse effects on normal cells. Vitamin E succinate enhanced the therapeutic efficacy, without any evidence of systemic toxicity, of a tolerated dose of calcitriol on prostate-cancer cells growing in athymic mice. Vitamin C in combination with lysine, proline, and green tea extract reduced the growth of a number of cancer cells in culture and in animals. A review of three studies revealed that vitamin C in combination with BCG produced beneficial effects in patients with bladder cancer and that vitamin E in combination with omega-3-fatty acids increased the survival of patients with advanced cancer (Coulter et al. 2006). Analysis of thirty-eight studies showed that vitamin C or vitamin E alone produced some beneficial effects on the survival of cancer patients (Coulter et al. 2006).

ENHANCING THE EFFICACY OF STANDARD THERAPY ON CANCER CELLS WITH THERAPEUTIC DOSES OF INDIVIDUAL ANTIOXIDANTS

The exact reasons why antioxidants increase the effectiveness of standard therapy on cancer cells are unknown. Based on the data discussed previously, treatment of tumors with therapeutic doses of antioxidants before standard therapy can initiate damage in cancer cells but not in normal cells. Cancer cells damaged by antioxidants continue to be treated with antioxidants and cancer-therapeutic agents that would kill more cancer cells than the individual agents alone. The damage to cancer cells produced by antioxidants may, in part, be different from that caused by standard therapeutic agents. Some of these differences are listed here.

1. Therapeutic doses of antioxidants, such as retinoic acid, can inhibit the repair of radiation damage in cancer cells more than in normal cells.

2. Vitamin E succinate–induced growth-inhibiting effects on cancer cells is not mediated by tumor-suppressor genes p53 and p21, whereas 5-FU-induced growth-inhibiting effects on cancer cells is mediated via p53 and p21. Therefore, the combination of two agents can be more effective than the individual agents.

3. Increased levels of the oncogenes c-myc and H-ras make cancer cells resistant to radiation, whereas vitamin E succinate treatment decreases the levels of these oncogenes in cancer cells. Therefore, the combination of radiation and vitamin E succinate can cause more cell death than the individual agents alone.

4. Vitamin E succinate and NAC act as anti-angiogenesis agents and thereby reduce the growth of tumor cells. Radiation- or chemotherapeutic agent–induced growth inhibition of cancer cells is not due to their anti-angiogenesis effect. Therefore, the combination of vitamin E succinate with these therapeutic agents can be more effective than the individual agents.

5. Antioxidants enhance damage to cancer cells caused by radiation or chemotherapeutic agents, but this may not be because of their antioxidant activity or because cancer cells accumulate more antioxidants than normal cells. It is possible that antioxidants alter gene expressions and cell-signaling systems that are

different from those produced by radiation and chemotherapeutic agents.

6. Antioxidant treatment may not initiate damage in normal cells before standard therapy. Therefore, when these cells are treated with radiation or chemotherapeutic agents, they can actually be protected by antioxidants through their classical antioxidant activity. On the other hand, therapeutic doses of antioxidants initiate damage in cancer cells before the standard therapy. When these damaged cancer cells are treated with standard treatment agents, there is further damage. In addition, continued treatment with antioxidants will continue to cause more damage.

RATIONALE FOR USING MULTIPLE MICRONUTRIENTS RATHER THAN A SINGLE ONE

We recommend the use of multiple micronutrients, including therapeutic doses of dietary antioxidants and coenzyme Q10, during cancer treatment with radiation therapy and/or chemotherapy. However, for cancer survivors, we recommend the use of multiple micronutrients containing preventive doses of dietary and endogenous antioxidants and coenzyme Q10. The scientific rationale for using multiple micronutrients is described here. The references for this section have been included in a review (Prasad 2011).

1. Several different types of free radicals are produced in the body, and each antioxidant has a different affinity for each of these, depending on the cellular environment.

2. Antioxidants produce different actions on cancer cells. For example, beta-carotene is more effective in quenching oxygen radicals than most other antioxidants, and it can perform certain biological functions that cannot be produced by vitamin A. On the other hand, vitamin A produces some effects that cannot be produced by beta-carotene. Also, beta-carotene treatment

increases the level of a gene called connexin (which produces a gap-junction protein that holds two normal cells together, a feature that can be lost in cancer cells), whereas vitamin A treatment does not. Vitamin A treatment induces differentiation in certain normal and cancer cells, whereas beta-carotene does not.

3. The levels of oxygen pressure vary within cells and tissues. Vitamin E is more effective as a quencher of free radicals in reduced oxygen pressure, whereas beta-carotene and vitamin A are more effective at a higher oxygen pressure.

4. Vitamin C is necessary to protect cellular components in water-soluble environments, whereas carotenoids and vitamins A and E protect cellular components in fat-soluble environments. More than 85 percent of the cellular environment contains water-soluble materials that are essential for the growth and survival of cells.

5. Vitamin C also plays an important role in maintaining cellular levels of vitamin E by recycling the vitamin E radical (oxidized) to the reduced (antioxidant) form.

6. The form and type of vitamin E used is also important in order to improve beneficial effects of vitamin E; vitamin E succinate is the most effective form. Therefore, both alpha-tocopherol or alpha-tocopheryl acetate and vitamin E succinate should be present in a multiple-micronutrient preparation.

7. Selenium, a cofactor of glutathione peroxidase, acts as an antioxidant. Selenium in combination with vitamin E succinate is more effective in reducing radiation-induced cancer formation in laboratory experiments than the individual agents alone. In addition, therapeutic doses of selenium can kill tumor cells without killing normal cells.

8. Glutathione, an endogenously made compound, represents a potent intracellular protective agent against oxidative damage. It catabolizes H_2O_2 and anions and is very effective in quenching peroxynitrite. Therefore, increasing the intracellular levels of glutathione may be important for maintaining good health. In

studies, oral supplementation with glutathione failed to significantly increase plasma levels of the tripeptide in human subjects, suggesting that it is completely degraded in the gastrointestinal tract. N-acetylcysteine and alpha-lipoic acid increase the intracellular levels of glutathione and, therefore, can also be used in combination with dietary antioxidants in a multiple-vitamin preparation.

9. Coenzyme Q10 is required for generating energy in the form of adenosine triphosphate (ATP) by mitochondria. Mitochondrial dysfunction that is associated with aging may mean that the mitochondria do not have adequate amounts of coenzyme Q10 to generate sufficient energy. Therefore, supplementation with coenzyme Q10 may be necessary for maintaining good health and for cancer prevention. In addition, coenzyme Q10 also scavenges peroxy radicals faster than alpha-tocopherol, and, like vitamin C, can regenerate vitamin E in a redox cycle.

10. All B vitamins are needed in a multiple-micronutrient preparation for optimal health.

RATIONALE FOR *NOT* RECOMMENDING ANTIOXIDANT SUPPLEMENTS DURING STANDARD THERAPY

At stated previously, most oncologists do not recommend antioxidants during radiation therapy or chemotherapy. There have been no clinical studies on the use of antioxidants during these therapies for cancer, but their recommendations are based primarily on laboratory experiments, some of which are described in the subsequent sections.

Increased Accumulation of Radioactive
Vitamin C in Tumor Cells Growing in Animals
The references for this section have been included in a review (Prasad 2011).

Some investigators have reported that therapeutic doses of vitamin C should not be given to cancer patients in conjunction with radiation therapy or chemotherapy, based on studies in which radioactive vitamin C accumulated more in tumor cells growing in animals than in the brain tissue of the same animals. It is an established fact that whenever radioactive vitamin C is used in research, the actual amount of vitamin C is extremely small. Therefore, it is possible that tumor tissue, which is rich in blood vessels, can accumulate more radioactive vitamin C than the brain, which has relatively fewer blood vessels. The researchers of this study suggested that vitamin C should not be used in patients who are undergoing radiation therapy or chemotherapy because it may protect cancer cells against radiation- and chemotherapeutic agent–induced damage. Such a recommendation has no scientific basis, because the investigators did not perform clinical studies in which vitamin C is combined with radiation therapy or chemotherapy.

Relying on Data Obtained from the Use of Preventive Doses of Individual Antioxidants in Combination with Cancer Therapeutic Agents

Several studies have shown that preventive doses of antioxidants do not affect the growth of cancer cells or normal cells. Treatment of cancer cells with such doses of individual antioxidants just one time shortly before administration of a therapeutic agent has been shown to decrease the effectiveness of the treatment agents. Laboratory studies show that vitamin E (alpha-tocopherol), vitamin C, or N-acetylcysteine (NAC), when given in a single preventive dose shortly before X-irradiation, decreases the effectiveness of irradiation on cancer cells. Treatment of leukemia and lymphoma cells in culture with preventive doses of vitamin C reduced the growth-inhibiting effect of doxorubicin, cisplatin, vincristine, and methotrexate. Preventive doses of vitamin C administered before doxorubicin treatment reduced therapeutic efficacy of this chemotherapy treatment in athymic mice with transplanted human lymphoma cells. Preventive doses of antioxidants used in these studies did not affect the growth of cancer cells. Alpha-lipoic acid at preventive doses reduced the effectiveness of doxorubicin in mouse leukemia. N-acetylcysteine at a preventive dose reduced cisplatin-induced cell killing from about 31 percent to about 11 percent in bladder-cancer cells. In our opinion the data obtained from the use of preventive doses of individual antioxidants in combination with radiation or chemotherapeutic agents should not be used to justify the avoidance of multiple micronutrients containing therapeutic doses of antioxidants.

We should point out that animal (primarily rats and mice) cancer cells show a high degree of resistance to most therapeutic agents when compared with normal cells. For example, anti-angiogenesis agents, amifostine, and proteasome inhibitors were found to be very effective in reducing the growth of tumor cells or in enhancing the effectiveness of therapeutic agents in animals. However, these agents even at lower doses were toxic to humans. The doses of antioxidants or drugs that are used in animal cancer-treatment studies should not be extrapolated to calculate the doses that would be relevant for human studies. Animal experiments are good for testing the potential value of antioxidants in the treatment of cancer. However, the data on doses obtained from animal studies may not be relevant to the treatment of human cancer.

Relying on Data Obtained from the use of Preventive Doses of Individual Antioxidants in Populations at High Risk of Developing Cancer

There are no cancer-treatment trials that indicate that therapeutic doses of multiple antioxidants (when given before therapy and every day thereafter for the entire treatment period) have ever reduced the efficacy of radiation therapy or chemotherapy. Often-quoted studies include those epidemiologic investigations or interventional trials that primarily use one antioxidant at preventive doses in high-risk populations (such as heavy tobacco smokers). For example, daily oral administration of synthetic beta-carotene (25 mg) revealed an increased incidence of lung cancer among male heavy smokers by 17 percent (The Alpha-tocopherol Beta-carotene Cancer Prevention Study Group 1994). These studies are often quoted as evidence for not recommending antioxidants during cancer therapy. Heavy smokers have a high oxidative environment in their bodies. Therefore, any single antioxidant, including beta-carotene, would be oxidized to form free radicals that can increase the risk of lung cancer.

An epidemiologic study analyzed ninety patients with breast cancer who took vitamin/mineral regimens within 180 days of diagnosis and continued them for a two-month period, whether or not they received radiation therapy, chemotherapy, or both (Seifried et al. 2003). These three treatment variables were separately grouped. However, the differences in treatments were not accounted for in data analysis. The above grouping of ninety patients into three treatment groups will yield only thirty patients per treatment group. Further variations in follow-up period and the doses, type, and number of micronutrients make it impossible to draw any reasonable conclusion regarding the effectiveness of micronutrient therapy. The variations in the experimental design of the above study are listed below.

Variations in follow-up period: Follow-up period varied from 20 months to 133 months, with a median value of 48 months. The study did not mention whether patients were taking vitamin/mineral during follow-up period.

Variations in doses and type of micronutrients: Beta-carotene doses varied from 0 to 250,000 IU, vitamin B_3 from 0 to greater than 1 mg, vitamin C from 1 to 24 g, selenium from 0 to 1,000 mcg, and zinc from 0 to greater than 50 mg.

Variations in number of micronutrients consumed by patients: Among 90 patients, 2 percent took three micronutrients, 23 percent took four micronutrients, 56 percent took five micronutrients, and 19 percent took all six micronutrients. In all cases no doses were given, and in the first four cases, the specific micronutrients were not named.

No meaningful conclusions regarding the value of micronutrients in breast-cancer treatment can be made based on this study, in which there were large variations in the follow-up period, doses, and type of micronutrients, and the number of micronutrients consumed by patients, while the number of patients in each treatment group was very small. Nevertheless, the authors concluded that breast cancer–specific survival and disease-free survival time was not improved by vitamin/mineral therapy. The patients taking vitamin/mineral supplements had poor survival and disease-free survival time in comparison to historical control receiving standard therapy. The publication that ran the study received wide publicity. However, the correct analysis of the data reveals that the flawed experimental design makes it impossible to base any recommendations on its results.

In another clinical trial 540 patients with stage I or II head and neck cancer received radiation therapy with a placebo or radiation therapy with synthetic vitamin E and beta-carotene at preventive doses (dl-alpha-tocopherol, 400 IU; beta-carotene, 30 mg) and were followed for three years. The beta-carotene supplementation was discontinued after 156 patients enrolled in the trial had concerns based on previous research in which beta-carotene alone at preventive doses increased the incidence of lung cancer by about 17 percent in male tobacco smokers. The remaining 384 patients continued to receive alpha-tocopherol alone. The results showed that supplementation with vitamin E among smokers enhanced the incidence of recurrence of primary tumors and death due to cancer or from all causes (Meyer et al. 2008).

Several issues can be raised with the design of the above clinical study. The preventive dose of vitamin E was used during radiation therapy, and preventive doses are known to decrease radiation-induced damage in both normal and cancer cells. This is not true with higher therapeutic doses of vitamin E (vitamin E succinate) or other antioxidants that selectively increase the growth-inhibiting effects of radiation on cancer cells but not on normal cells. Unfortunately, the authors concluded, "Particular attention should be devoted to prevent patients from smoking and taking antioxidant supplements during radiation therapy."

Relying on Data Obtained from Antioxidant Deficiency in Combination with Therapeutic Agents in Cancer Cells

Certain amounts of micronutrients, including antioxidants, are needed for the survival and growth of cancer cells. Therefore, antioxidant deficiency will reduce the growth of cancer cells. Indeed, it has been reported that a diet deficient in vitamins A and E increases cell killing in brain tumors growing in transgenic mice (those genetically engineered to develop brain tumors) by about fivefold. It also reduces tumor size by about 50 percent after four months on the vitamin-deficient diet, in comparison to a standard diet or a diet rich in vitamins A and E (twofold more than that in standard diet). No evidence of adverse effects in the spleen, small intestine, or liver were found. From these results, some researchers inferred that if the deficiency of antioxidants reduces the growth of cancer cells, then an excess of them may increase their growth. This inference, however, is not applicable to therapeutic doses of dietary antioxidants, which cause growth inhibition in cancer cells without affecting most normal cells. It should also be pointed out that a deficiency in vitamins A and E may induce irreversible neurological and neuromuscular damage and other toxicities. Furthermore, such an antioxidant-deficient diet before treatment may enhance the effect of X-irradiation or chemotherapeutic agents on both cancer cells and normal cells. Antioxidant deficiency by itself may cause irreversible neurological damage in humans. Therefore, creating an antioxidant deficiency before standard therapy may not be a useful cancer-treatment strategy.

ENHANCEMENT OF THE BENEFICIAL EFFECTS OF EXPERIMENTAL THERAPEUTIC AGENTS WITH THERAPEUTIC DOSES OF ANTIOXIDANTS

Hyperthermia (Heat Therapy)

The references for this section have been included in a review (Prasad 2011).

Heat therapy is designed to kill cancer cells without killing normal cells. Hyperthermia at 42° to 43°C (107.6 to 109.4°F) alone, or in combination with radiation, is primarily used in the management of local tumors when all other therapeutic modalities have failed. This approach has not been effective for the long-term management of tumors. Therefore, the treatment may need to be altered from local hyperthermia at higher temperatures to whole-body hyperthermia at lower temperatures that could be tolerated without side effects. In addition, therapeutic doses of antioxidants could be used to enhance the effectiveness of hyperthermia on cancer cells. Our laboratory research has shown that vitamin E succinate markedly increases the growth-inhibiting effect of low temperature (41°C) and high temperature (43°C) on neuroblastoma cells in culture (see Table 8.6). Administration of vitamin C locally into the tumor greatly enhances the efficacy of hyperthermia in reducing the growth of lung carcinoma in mice. Therapeutic doses of vitamin C in combination with hyperthermia increase the survival time of mice carrying Ehrlich ascites mammary carcinoma cells, compared to untreated control animals. Other groups of antioxidants, such as the bioflavonoid quercetin, in combination with hyperthermia cause synergistic cell death in lymphoid-cancer cells in culture. Quercetin and tamoxifen together enhance hyperthermia-induced cell killing in a synergistic manner in human melanoma cells in culture. Quercetin may also be useful in increasing the tumor responses to hyperthermia in combination chemotherapy. We propose that oral administration of therapeutic doses of multiple micronutrients in combination with hyperthermia delivered locally to the tumor (42 to 43°C) or to the whole body (40°C, or 104°F) may further improve the effectiveness of hyperthermia in the treatment of human cancer.

TABLE 8.6. EFFECT OF ALPHA-TOCOPHERYL SUCCINATE (VITAMIN E SUCCINATE) ON HYPERTHERMIA-INDUCED GROWTH INHIBITION IN NEUROBLASTOMA CELLS IN CULTURE

Treatments	Cell Number (Percent of Controls)
Solvent (ethanol 0.25 percent) +	
Sodium succinate (5 µg/ml)	102 ± 3
Vitamin E succinate (5 µg /ml)	50 ± 3
43°C (20 min)	43 ± 1
Vitamin E succinate + 43°C	9 ± 1
41°C (45 min)	56 ± 3
Vitamin E succinate + 41°C	21 ± 2
40°C (8 hr)	55 ± 2
Vitamin E succinate + 40°C	30 ± 2

Average value ± SEM (standard error of the mean)
µg = micrograms
µL = milliliter

From K. N. Prasad, *Micronutrients In Health and Disease,* Boca Raton, Fla.: Francis and Taylor Publishing Groups, 2011.

Vitamin E succinate treatment enhanced the growth-inhibiting effect of heat therapy on cancer cells.

Sodium Butyrate

Butyric acid, a four-carbon fatty acid, is formed in the colon by the combination of fiber and beneficial bacteria that are present in the lower colon. Our laboratory research has shown that sodium butyrate inhibits the growth of cancer cells without affecting the growth of normal cells. Sodium butyrate is rapidly degraded in the body; therefore, a derivative of butyric acid, phenylbutyrate, was developed. Treatment with phenylbutyrate causes cell killing and growth inhibition in several animal and human tumor cells in culture. However, in clinical studies oral administration of therapeutic doses of sodium butyrate or phenylbutyrate produced minimal benefits in cancer patients (Thibault et al. 2009). Therefore, any agents that can enhance the effectiveness of sodium butyrate or phenylbutyrate would enhance the value of these agents in the management of human cancers. Our laboratory research has shown that vitamin E succinate at therapeutic doses enhances the growth-inhibiting effect of sodium butyrate on certain tumor cells in culture. Retinoic acid also increases the effectiveness of phenylbutyrate-induced growth inhibition on human prostate-cancer cells and reduces angiogenesis in athymic mice. Retinoic acid in combination with sodium butyrate also caused a synergistic effect on cell differentiation in highly malignant thyroid-cancer cells in culture; however, in athymic mice carrying the same tumor, the combination of two agents did not reduce the growth of tumor more than that produced by retinoic acid treatment alone. This may be because sodium butyrate is rapidly degraded in the body. Laboratory research has shown that antioxidants such as quercetin, curcumin, and ferulic acid enhance sodium butyrate–induced cell killing in human leukemia cells in culture.

Interferon Alpha-2a

Interferon alpha-2a is produced by the immune cells. It inhibits the growth of cancer cells. Laboratory research has shown that retinoic acid enhances the growth-inhibiting effect of interferon alpha-2a on squamous-cell carcinoma of the cervix. Although treatment of squamous-cell carcinoma of the head and neck with retinoic acid, interferon alpha-2a, and vitamin E succinate individually or in a dual combination produced varying degree of growth inhibition, the combination of all three was most effective. The combination of 13-cis-retinoic acid and interferon alpha-2a enhanced radiation-induced growth inhibition in human cervical-carcinoma cells in culture.

Cellular Vaccine

Dendritic cells are potential candidates for immunotherapy, because they have the ability to process and present antigens to T-cell lymphocytes and increase the immune responses that can kill cancer cells. This therapy has exhibited minimal antitumor activity in established tumors in mice and humans. Vitamin E succinate administered locally or systemically has been reported to enhance the effectiveness of dendritic cells injected intratumorally or subcutaneously in reducing the size of tumors in mice. Vesiculated vitamin E succinate, a more soluble form of vitamin E succinate, is equally effective in reducing the growth of tumor cells. This form of vitamin E succinate in combination with dendritic cells is more effective in reducing the growth of tumor cells than vesiculated vitamin E succinate alone. Vitamin E succinate in combination with tumor necrosis factor–related apoptosis-inducing ligand (TRAIL), a potential chemotherapeutic agent, and dendritic cells caused a marked tumor-growth inhibition or induced a complete tumor regression.

Gene Therapy
Adenovirus-mediated mda-7 (Ad-mda) gene transfer has been shown to induce cell killing in various human cancer cells without killing normal cells. Vitamin E succinate also produces similar effects on normal and cancer cells. Treatment of human ovarian cells in culture with Ad-mda and vitamin E succinate induced cell killing more than that produced by the individual agents; however, it did not affect the growth of normal cells.

Proposed Micronutrient Preparations in Cancer Treatment
Based on the extensive laboratory studies and some human studies presented in this chapter, we propose three distinct multiple-micronutrient preparations: (1) one that is used in combination with standard therapy, (2) one that is used in cancer patients who have become unresponsive to all therapies, and (3) one that is used in survivors after completion of cancer therapy. These proposed micronutrient preparations, together with changes in diet and lifestyle, should be adopted in consultation with a physician, with the goal of improving clinical outcomes in each group of patients.

Ingredients of a Multiple-Micronutrient Preparation in Combination with Standard Therapy
Based on new laboratory and some clinical studies, we propose a modification to our original micronutrient preparation published in the 2001 edition of this book. The modified multiple micronutrient preparation contains:

- vitamin A, 10,000 IU
- vitamin C, 5 g
- d-alpha-tocopheryl succinate, 1,600 IU
- natural carotenoids, 100 mg
- selenomethionine, 200 mcg
- coenzyme Q10, 200 mg
- omega-3 fatty acids, 4 g
- vitamin D, 1,000 IU
- B vitamins, two to three times higher than RDA values
- appropriate minerals

This formulation does not contain glutathione-elevating agents (n-acetylcysteine and alpha-lipoic acid), because high levels of glutathione in the cells may protect both cancer cells and normal cells against therapeutic agents. This formulation can be administered orally in two doses, one in the morning and one in the evening with a meal. The rate of elimination of micronutrients from the body varies; therefore, taking these micronutrients twice a day maintains their high levels. The micronutrient preparation should be administered at least three days prior to standard or experimental therapy and should be continued daily for the entire period of treatment and for an additional one month after the completion of therapy. Ideally, the micronutrient preparation will improve the effectiveness of radiation therapy and/or chemotherapy by increasing tumor-cell killing without enhancing normal-cell killing and possibly decrease toxicity. It should not be used before surgery, because high doses of vitamin E may interfere with blood clotting; however, it can be administered two days after surgery in order to help with the healing process.

A phase-I study, followed by a well-designed clinical study, is needed in order to determine the safety of the proposed micronutrient protocol. The results obtained from these studies would help settle the current controversies and may markedly enhance the effectiveness of standard and experimental cancer therapies.

Ingredients of a Multiple-Micronutrient Preparation for Patients Who Have Become Unresponsive to All Therapies

At present, there are no effective strategies to enhance the survival time with a good quality of life for patients who have become unresponsive to all standard and experimental therapies. These patients often die within a few months, in spite of current supportive care. The use of a multiple-micronutrient preparation in combination with supportive care may prolong the survival time with an improved quality of life. This multiple-micronutrient preparation contains:

- vitamin A, 10,000 IU
- vitamin C, 10 g
- d-alpha-tocopheryl succinate, 1,600 IU
- natural carotenoids, 100 mg
- selenomethionine, 300 mcg
- coenzyme Q10, 400 mg
- n-acetyl-cysteine (NAC), 500 mg
- alpha-lipoic acid, 400 mg
- omega-3 fatty acids, 4 g
- vitamin D, 1,000 IU
- B vitamins, two to three times higher than RDA values
- appropriate minerals

This formulation can be administered orally in two doses, one in the morning and one in the evening with a meal. The rate of elimination of micronutrients from the body varies; therefore, taking these micronutrients twice a day will maintain their high levels. The micronutrient preparation should be administered when all therapies have failed and should be continued daily for the entire life span. This preparation has the goal of improving the survival time and improving quality of life by limiting the growth of tumors and improving overall well-being.

Ingredients of a Multiple-Micronutrient
Preparation for Cancer Survivors

As discussed previously, cancer survivors have increased risk of recurrence of the primary tumor, as well as the development of new cancers. At present there is no effective strategy to reduce the recurrence of tumors, except in the case of low-dose tamoxifen for breast cancer. Some adverse health effects, such as high levels of lipids in the blood and increased risk of stroke, have been observed in breast-cancer patients taking tamoxifen. Antioxidant supplementation appears to decrease these side effects. We propose that one month after completion of standard therapy, the following preventive-dose micronutrient preparation be started. This formulation contains:

- vitamin A, 3,000 IU
- vitamin C, 1,500 mg
- vitamin E, 400 IU (300 IU d-alpha-tocopheryl succinate and 100 IU alpha-tocopheryl acetate)
- selenomethionine, 100 mcg
- coenzyme Q10, 60 mg
- alpha-lipoic acid, 60 mg
- n-acetylcysteine, 250 mg
- L-carnitine, 150 mg
- vitamin D, 800 IU
- B vitamins, two to three times higher than RDA values
- appropriate minerals, but no iron, copper, or manganese

This patented formulation is available commercially as Cellular Security (www.mypmcinside.com) and can be started at any time after therapy. The goal is to reduce the recurrence of the primary tumor, improve quality of life, and reduce the risk of developing secondary new tumors.

RECOMMENDATIONS FOR DIET
AND LIFESTYLE CHANGES

Diet and lifestyle changes should be adopted by all three groups of cancer patients and are equally important in improving the efficacy of the proposed micronutrient preparation. We recommend a diet low in fat, high in fiber, and rich in fresh fruits and vegetables. We also recommend reducing intake of nitrite-rich food, such as bacon, sausage, and cured luncheon meat. Recommended changes in lifestyle include stopping the use of tobacco and tobacco products, reduced physical and mental stress, moderate daily exercise, avoidance of excessive caffeine and alcoholic beverages, and reduced exposure to the sun and UV light.

CONCLUDING REMARKS

The incidence of cancer is on the rise and overall cancer mortality remains high. Cancer patients can be divided into three groups: (a) those receiving standard or experimental therapy, (b) those who become unresponsive to these therapies, and (c) those in remission who have the risk of recurrence of primary tumors or the development of secondary new cancers. While progress in standard cancer therapy has been made, the value of this therapy in the management of solid tumors may have reached a plateau. In addition, adverse serious side effects during and after therapy remain a major concern. At present there is no effective strategy for improving the effectiveness of standard therapy, improving the survival time of patients who have become unresponsive to all therapies, or reducing the risk of recurrence of primary tumors or the development of secondary new cancers among survivors. Therefore, additional approaches should be developed to improve clinical outcomes in all these groups of cancer patients. The goal of our proposed micronutrient preparations is to improve health in all three groups.

At present most oncologists do not recommend antioxidant supplements during radiation therapy or chemotherapy for fear that they may reduce the effectiveness of the therapy. On the other hand, many cancer patients take antioxidant supplements without the knowledge of their oncologists. There is a great deal of controversy not only between patients and oncologists but also between nutritional oncology researchers and clinicians. The major reasons include: (a) failure to distinguish between the effects of preventive and therapeutic doses of antioxidants alone or in combination with therapeutic agents on cancer cells, (b) failure to appreciate the selective-killing effect of therapeutic doses of antioxidants on cancer cells but not on normal cells, (c) the assumption that the effect of a single antioxidant in clinical studies would be similar to those produced by a multiple-vitamin preparation containing therapeutic doses of antioxidants, and (d) relying on data obtained from the use of a single antioxidant in prevention studies. Resolving these controversies is important for researchers and cancer patients.

This chapter has presented experimental and clinical results on the effects of antioxidants alone or in combination with ionizing radiation and chemotherapeutic agents on both cancer cells and normal cells. From the critical analysis of these data, it appears that therapeutic doses of antioxidants inhibit the growth of cancer cells without affecting the growth of normal cells. They also increased the growth-inhibiting effects of therapeutic agents on cancer cells while protecting normal cells against some types of damage. On the other hand, preventive doses of antioxidants have no effect on, or in some cases may enhance the growth of, cancer cells. Preventive doses of antioxidants can also reduce the growth-inhibiting effect of standard therapeutic agents.

Based on extensive laboratory studies and some human studies with therapeutic doses of antioxidants alone or in combination with radiation therapy and/or chemotherapy, we propose three distinct multiple micronutrient preparations: (1) one that should be used in combination with standard therapy, (2) one that should be used in cancer patients who have become unresponsive to all therapies, and (3) one that should be used in survivors after completion of cancer therapy. These proposed micronutrient preparations, together with changes in diet and lifestyle, should be adopted in consultation with a physician in order to improve the clinical outcomes for each group of patients.

9 Values of Recommended Daily Allowances (RDA)/ Dietary Reference Intakes (DRI)

Sufficient changes in nutritional guidelines have occurred since World War II, in keeping with increased knowledge of nutrition and health. The nutritional guidelines referred to as Recommended Daily Allowances (RDAs) were first established in 1941. The Food and Nutrition Board of the United States revises these guidelines every five to ten years.

RDA (DRI)

RDA refers to the value of the daily dietary intake of a nutrient considered sufficient to meet the requirements of 97 to 98 percent of healthy individuals of different ages and genders. Because of rapid growth of research on the role of nutrients in human health, the Food and Nutrition Board of the Institute of Medicine (IOM) of the United States, in collaboration with Health Canada, updated the values of RDAs and renamed them Dietary Reference Intakes (DRIs) in 1998. The DRI values of selected nutrients are listed in Tables 9.1 to 9.21. The DRI values are not currently used in nutrition labeling; RDA values continue to be used for this purpose. The

DRI values for carotenoids, alpha-lipoic acid, N-acetylcysteine, coenzyme Q10, and L-carnitine have not been determined.

ADEQUATE INTAKE (AI)

AI refers to the value of a nutrient for which no RDA has been established, but the value established may be sufficient for everyone in the demographic group.

TOLERABLE UPPER INTAKE LEVEL (UL)

This is the maximum level of daily nutrient intake that is likely to pose no risk of adverse health effects. The UL value represents the total intake of a nutrient from food, water, and supplements.

RELATIONSHIP BETWEEN RECOMMENDED DAILY ALLOWANCES AND HEALTH

RDA values of nutrients are expected to be adequate for individuals for normal growth and survival; however, the values of micronutrients needed for prevention or improved management of human diseases are not known at this time. The data on doses obtained from the use of a single micronutrient in the prevention or treatment of human cancer should not be extrapolated to the doses of the same micronutrient when part of a multiple-micronutrient preparation. Generally, whenever a single micronutrient is used in the laboratory to evaluate its growth-inhibiting effect on cancer cells, therapeutic doses that do not affect the growth of normal cells are needed to observe this effect.

Preventive doses of the same micronutrient do not inhibit the growth of cancer cells or normal cells. Low preventive doses may even stimulate the growth of some cancer cells. Therefore, it is essential that the distinction between the effects of preventive doses and therapeutic doses of antioxidants is made while evaluating their effectiveness in cancer prevention and treatment. In order to evaluate the dosage of micronutrients in any multiple-vitamin preparation for the prevention or treatment of cancer, it is essential to have sufficient knowledge of the RDA values of the micronutrients.

TABLE 9.1. DIETARY REFERENCE INTAKES (DRI) OF ANTIOXIDANT VITAMIN A

Age	RDA/AI*	UL
	µg/d (IU/d)	µg/d (IU/d)
Infants		
0–6 mo	400 (1,200 IU)*	600 (1,800 IU)
7–12 mo	500 (1,500 IU)*	600 (1,800 IU)
Children		
1–3 y	300 (900 IU)	600 (1,800 IU)
4–8 y	400 (1,200 IU)	900 (2,700 IU)
Males		
9–13 y	600 (1,800 IU)	1,700 (5,100 IU)
14–18 y	900 (2,700 IU)	2,800 (8,400 IU)
19 y and up	900 (2,700 IU)	3,000 (9,000 IU)
Females		
9–13 y	600 (1,800 IU)	1,700 (5,100 IU)
14–18 y	700 (2,100 IU)	2,800 (8,400 IU)
19 y and up	700 (2,100 IU)	3,000 (9,000 IU)
Pregnancy		
under 18 y	750 (2,250 IU)	2,800 (8,400 IU)
19–50 y	770 (2310 IU)	3,000 (9,000 IU)
Lactation		
under 18 y	1,200 (3,600 IU)	2,800 (8,400 IU)
19–50 y	1,300 (3,900 IU)	3,000 (9,000 IU)

1 µg of retinol equals 1µg of RAE (retinol activity equivalent); 1 IU of retinol equals 0.3 µg of retinol; and 2 µg of beta-carotene equals 1 µg of retinol.

RDA = Recommended Daily Allowance
*AI = Adequate Intake
UL = Tolerable Upper Intake Value
µg = microgram; d = day

The values are adapted and summarized from the table of the Dietary Reference Intakes (DRI) published by www.nap.edu. (Search on "Food and Nutrition" and you will find Information about DRI.)

TABLE 9.2. DIETARY REFERENCE INTAKES (DRI) OF ANTIOXIDANT VITAMIN C

Age	RDA/AI*	UL
	mg/d	mg/d
Infants		
0–6 mo	40*	ND
7–12 mo	50*	ND
Children		
1–3 y	15	400
4–8 y	25	650
Males		
9–13 y	45	1,200
14–18 y	75	1, 800
19 y and up	90	2,000
Females		
9–13 y	45	1,200
14–18 y	65	1,800
19 y and up	75	2,000

RDA = Recommended Daily Allowance
*AI = Adequate Intake
UL = Tolerable Upper Intake Value
µg = microgram; d = day

The values are adapted and summarized from the table of the Dietary Reference Intakes (DRI) published by www.nap.edu.

TABLE 9.3. DIETARY REFERENCE INTAKES (DRI) OF ANTIOXIDANT VITAMIN E

Age	RDA/AI*	UL
	mg/d (IU/d)	mg/d (IU/d)
Infants		
0–6 mo	4 (6 IU)*	ND
7–12 mo	5 (7.5 IU)*	ND
Children		
1–3 y	6 (9 IU)	200 (30 IU)
4–8 y	7 (10.6 IU)	300 (45 IU)
Males		
9–13 y	11 (16.7 IU)	600 (90 IU)
14–18 y	15 (22.8 IU)	800 (120 IU)
19 y and up	15 (22.8 IU)	1,000 (150 IU)
Females		
9–13 y	11 (16.7 IU)	600 (90 IU)
14–18 y	15 (22.8 IU)	800 (120 IU)
19 y and up	15 (22.8 IU)	1,000 (150 IU)
Pregnancy		
under 18 y	15 (22.8 IU)	800 (120 IU)
19–50 y	15 (22.8 IU)	1,000 (150 IU)
Lactation		
under 18 y	19 (28.9 IU)	800 (120 IU)
19–50 y	19 (28.9 IU)	1,000 (150 IU)

RDA = Recommended Daily Allowance
*AI = Adequate Intake
UL = Tolerable Upper Intake Value
ND = not determined
mg = milligram; d = day
1 IU of vitamin E equals 0.66 mg of d- and 0.45 mg of
dl-alpha-tocopherol

The values are adapted and summarized from the tables of the Dietary Reference Intakes (DRI) published by www.nap.edu.

TABLE 9.4. DIETARY REFERENCE INTAKES (DRI) OF VITAMIN D

Age	RDA/AI*	UL
	µg/d (IU/d)	µg/d (IU/d)
Infants		
0–12 mo	5 (200 IU)*	25 (1,000 IU)
Children		
1–8 y	5 (200 IU)*	50 (2,000 IU)
Males		
9–50 y	5 (200 IU)*	50 (2,000 IU)
50–70 y	10 (400 IU)*	50 (2,000 IU)
over 70 y	15 (600 IU)*	50 (2,000 IU)
Females		
9–50 y	5 (200 IU)*	50 (2,000 IU)
50–70 y	10 (400 IU)*	50 (2,000 IU)
under 70 y	15 (600 IU)*	50 (2,000 IU)
Pregnancy		
18–50 y	5 (200 IU)*	50 (2,000 IU)
Lactation		
18–50 y	5 (200 IU)*	50 (2,000 IU)

RDA = Recommended Daily Allowance
*AI = Adequate Intake
UL = Tolerable Upper Intake Value
µg = microgram; d = day
1 µg of cholecalciferol equals 40 IU (international unit)
of Vitamin D.

The values are adapted and summarized from the tables of the Dietary Reference Intakes (DRI) published by www.nap.edu.

TABLE 9.5. DIETARY REFERENCE INTAKES (DRI) OF VITAMIN B$_1$ (THIAMINE)

Age	RDA/AI*	UL
	mg/d	mg/d
Infants		
0–6 mo	0.2*	ND
7–12 mo	0.3*	ND
Children		
1–3 y	0.5	ND
4–8 y	0.6	ND
Males		
9–13 y	0.9	ND
14 y and up	1.2	ND
Females		
9–13 y	0.9	ND
14–18 y	1.0	ND
19 y and up	1.1	ND
Pregnancy		
18–50 y	1.4	ND
Lactation		
18–50 y	1.4	ND

RDA = Recommended Daily Allowance
*AI = Adequate Intake
UL = Tolerable Upper Intake Value
ND = not determined
mg = milligram; d = day

The values are adapted and summarized from the tables of the Dietary Reference Intakes (DRI) published by www.nap.edu.

TABLE 9.6. DIETARY REFERENCE
INTAKES (DRI) OF VITAMIN B₂ (RIBOFLAVIN)

Age	RDA/AI*	UL
	mg/d	mg/d
Infants		
0–6 mo	0.3*	ND
7–12 mo	0.4*	ND
Children		
1–3 y	0.5	ND
4–8 y	0.6	ND
Males		
9–13 y	0.9	ND
14 y and up	13	ND
Females		
9–13	0.9	ND
14–18 y	1.0	ND
19 y and up	1.1	ND
Pregnancy		
18–50 y	1.4	ND
Lactation		
18–50 y	1.6	ND

RDA = Recommended Daily Allowance
*AI = Adequate Intake
UL = Tolerable Upper Intake Value
ND = not determined
mg = milligram; d = day

The values are adapted and summarized from the table of the Dietary Reference Intakes (DRI) published by www.nap.edu.

TABLE 9.7. DIETARY REFERENCE INTAKES (DRI) OF VITAMIN B₆

Age	RDA/AI*	UL
	mg/d	mg/d
Infants		
0–6 mo	0.1*	ND
7–12 mo	0.3*	ND
Children		
1–3 y	0.5	30
4–8 y	0.6	40
Males		
9–13 y	1.0	60
14–50 y	1.3	80
50–70 y and up	1.7	100
Females		
9–13 y	1.0	60
14–18 y	1.2	80
19–30 y	1.3	100
50 y and up	1.5	100
Pregnancy		
under 18 y	1.9	80
19–50 y	1.9	100
Lactation		
under 18 y	2.0	80
19–50 y	2.0	100

RDA = Recommended Daily Allowance
*AI = Adequate Intake
UL = Tolerable Upper Intake Value
ND = not determined
mg = milligram; d = day

The values are adapted and summarized from the table of the Dietary Reference Intakes (DRI) published by www.nap.edu.

TABLE 9.8. DIETARY REFERENCE
INTAKES (DRI) OF VITAMIN B₁₂ (COBALAMIN)

Age	RDA/AI*	UL
	µg/d	µg/d
Infants		
0–6 mo	0.4*	ND
7–12 mo	0.5*	ND
Children		
1–3 y	0.9	ND
4–8 y	1.2	ND
Males		
9–13 y	1.08	ND
14 y and up	2.4	ND
Females		
9–13 y	1.8	ND
14 y and up	2.4	ND
Pregnancy		
18–50 y	2.6	ND
Lactation		
18–50 y	2.8	ND

RDA = Recommended Daily Allowance
*AI = Adequate Intake
UL = Tolerable Upper Intake Value
ND = not determined
µg = microgram; d = day

The values are adapted and summarized from the table of the Dietary Reference Intakes (DRI) published by www.nap.edu.

TABLE 9.9. DIETARY REFERENCE
INTAKES (DRI) OF VITAMIN PANTOTHENIC ACID

Age	RDA/AI*	UL
	mg/d	mg/d
Infants		
0–6 mo	1.7*	ND
7–12 mo	1.8*	ND
Children		
1–3 y	2*	ND
4–8 y	2*	ND
Males		
9–13 y	4*	ND
14 y and up	5*	ND
Females		
9–13 y	4*	ND
14 y and up	5*	ND
Pregnancy		
18–50 y	6*	ND
Lactation		
18–50 y	7*	ND

RDA = Recommended Daily Allowance
*AI = Adequate Intake
UL = Tolerable Upper Intake Value
ND = not determined
mg = milligram; d = day

The values are adapted and summarized from the table of the Dietary Reference Intakes (DRI) published by www.nap.edu.

TABLE 9.10. DIETARY REFERENCE INTAKES (DRI) OF VITAMIN NIACIN

Age	RDA/AI*	UL
	mg/d	mg/d
Infants		
0–6 mo	2*	ND
7–12 mo	0.4*	ND
Children		
1–3 y	6.0	10
4–8 y	8.0	15
Males		
9–13 y	12	20
14–50 y	16	30
50 y and up	16	35
Females		
9–13 y	12	20
14–18 y	14	30
19 y and up	14	35
Pregnancy		
under 18 y	18	30
19–50 y	18	35
Lactation		
under 18 y	17	30
19–50 y	17	35

RDA = Recommended Daily Allowance
*AI = Adequate Intake
UL = Tolerable Upper Intake Value
ND = not determined
mg = milligram; d = day

The values are adapted and summarized from the table of the Dietary Reference Intakes (DRI) published by www.nap.edu

TABLE 9.11. DIETARY REFERENCE INTAKES (DRI) OF VITAMIN FOLATE

Age	RDA/AI*	UL
	µg/d	µg/d
Infants		
0–6 mo	65*	ND
7–12 mo	80*	ND
Children		
1–3 y	150	300
4–8 y	200	400
Males		
9–13 y	300	600
14–18 y	400	800
19 y and up	400	1,000
Females		
9–13 y	300	600
14–18 y	400	800
19 y and up	400	1,000
Pregnancy		
under 18 y	600	800
19–50 y	600	1,000
Lactation		
under 18 y	500	800
19–50 y	500	1,000

RDA = Recommended Daily Allowance
*AI = Adequate Intake
UL = Tolerable Upper Intake Value
ND = not determined
µg = microgram; d = day

The values are adapted and summarized from the table of the Dietary Reference Intakes (DRI) published by www.nap.edu.

TABLE 9.12. DIETARY REFERENCE INTAKES (DRI) OF MICRONUTRIENT BIOTIN

Age	RDA/AI*	UL
	µg/d	µg/d
Infants		
0–6 mo	0.5*	ND
7–12 mo	0.6*	ND
Children		
1–3 y	8*	ND
4–8 y	12*	ND
Males		
9–13 y	20	ND
14–18 y	25	ND
19 y and up	30	ND
Females		
9–13 y	20	ND
14–18 y	25	ND
19 y and up	30	ND
Pregnancy		
under 18 y	30*	ND
19–50 y	30*	ND
Lactation		
under 18 y	35*	ND
19–50 y	35*	ND

RDA = Recommended Daily Allowance
*AI = Adequate Intake
UL = Tolerable Upper Intake Value
ND = not determined
µg = microgram; d = day

The values are adapted and summarized from the table of the Dietary Reference Intakes (DRI) published by www.nap.edu.

TABLE 9.13. DIETARY REFERENCE INTAKES (DRI) OF MINERAL CALCIUM

Age	RDA/AI*	UL
	mg/d	mg/d
Infants		
0–6 mo	210*	ND
7–12 mo	270*	ND
Children		
1–3 y	500*	2,500
4–8 y	800*	2,500
Males		
9–18 y	1,300*	2,500
19–50 y	1,000*	2,500
51 y and up	1,200*	2,500
Females		
9–8 y	1,300*	2,500
19–50 y	1,000*	2,500
51 y and up	1,200*	2,500
Pregnancy		
under 18 y	1,300*	2,500
19–50 y	1,000*	2,500
Lactation		
under 18 y	1,300*	2,500
19–50 y	1,000*	2,500

RDA = Recommended Daily Allowance
*AI = Adequate Intake
UL = Tolerable Upper Intake Value
ND = not determined
mg = milligram; d = day

The values are adapted and summarized from the table of the Dietary Reference Intakes (DRI) published by www.nap.edu.

TABLE 9.14. DIETARY REFERENCE INTAKES (DRI) OF MINERAL MAGNESIUM

Age	RDA/AI*	UL
	mg/d	mg/d
Infants		
0–6 mo	30*	ND
7–12 mo	75*	ND
Children		
1–3 y	80	65
4–8 y	130	110
Males		
9–13 y	240	350
14–18 y	410	350
19–30 y	400	350
31 y and up	420	350
Females		
9–13 y	240	350
14–18 y	360	350
31 y and up	320	350
Pregnancy		
under 18 y	400	350
19–30 y	350	350
31–50 y	360	350
Lactation		
under 18 y	360	350
31–50 y	320	350

RDA = Recommended Daily Allowance
*AI = Adequate Intake
UL = Tolerable Upper Intake Value
ND = not determined
mg = milligram; d = day

The values are adapted and summarized from the table of the Dietary Reference Intakes (DRI) published by www.nap.edu.

TABLE 9.15. DIETARY REFERENCE INTAKES (DRI) OF MINERAL MANGANESE

Age	RDA/AI*	UL
	mg/d	mg/d
Infants		
0–6 mo	0.003*	ND
7–12 mo	0.6*	ND
Children		
1–3 y	1.2 *	2
4–8 y	1.5*	3
Males		
9–13 y	1.9*	6
14–18 y	2.2*	9
19 y and up	2.3*	11
Females		
9–13 y	1.6*	6
14–18 y	1.6 *	9
19 y and up	1.8*	11
Pregnancy		
under 18 y	2.0*	9
19–50 y	2.0*	11
Lactation		
under 18 y	2.6*	9
19–50 y	2.6*	11

RDA = Recommended Daily Allowance
*AI = Adequate Intake
UL = Tolerable Upper Intake Value
ND = not determined
mg = milligram; d = day

The values are adapted and summarized from the table of the Dietary Reference Intakes (DRI) published by www.nap.edu.

TABLE 9.16. DIETARY REFERENCE INTAKES (DRI) OF MINERAL CHROMIUM

Age	RDA/AI*	UL
	µg/d	µg/d
Infants		
0–6 mo	0.2*	ND
7–12 mo	5.5*	ND
Children		
1–3 y	11*	ND
4–8 y	15*	ND
Males		
9–13 y	25*	ND
14–50 y	35*	ND
51 y and up	30*	ND
Females		
9–13 y	21*	ND
14–18 y	24*	ND
19–50 y	25*	ND
Pregnancy		
under 18 y	29*	ND
19–50 y	30*	ND
Lactation		
under 18 y	44*	ND
19–50 y	45*	ND

RDA = Recommended Daily Allowance
*AI = Adequate Intake
UL = Tolerable Upper Intake Value
ND = not determined
µg = microgram; d = day

The values are adapted and summarized from the table of the Dietary Reference Intakes (DRI) published by www.nap.edu.

TABLE 9.17. DIETARY REFERENCE INTAKES (DRI) OF MINERAL COPPER

Age	RDA/AI*	UL
	µg/d	µg/d
Infants		
0–6 mo	200*	ND
7–12 mo	220*	ND
Children		
1–3 y	340	1,000
4–8 y	440	3,000
Males		
9–13 y	700	5,000
14–18 y	890	8,000
19 y and up	900	10,000
Females		
9–13 y	700	5,000
14–18 y	890	8,000
19 y and up	900	10,000
Pregnancy		
under 18 y	1,000	8,000
19–50 y	1,000	10,000
Lactation		
under 18 y	1,300	8,000
19–50 y	1,300	10,000

RDA = Recommended Daily Allowance
*AI = Adequate Intake
UL = Tolerable Upper Intake Value
ND = not determined
µg = microgram; d = day

The values are adapted and summarized from the table of the Dietary Reference Intakes (DRI) published by www.nap.edu.

TABLE 9.18. DIETARY REFERENCE INTAKES (DRI) OF MINERAL IRON

Age	RDA/AI*	UL
	mg/d	mg/d
Infants		
0–6 mo	0.27*	40
7–12 mo	11	40
Children		
1–3 y	7	40
4–8 y	10	40
Males		
9–13 y	8	40
14–18 y	11	45
19 y and up	8	45
Females		
9–13 y	8	40
14–18 y	15	45
19–50 y	18	45
50 y and up	8	45
Pregnancy		
18–50 y	27	45
Lactation		
under 18 y	10	45
19–50 y	9	45

RDA = Recommended Daily Allowance
*AI = Adequate Intake
UL = Tolerable Upper Intake Value
ND = not determined
mg = milligram; d = day

The values are adapted and summarized from the table of the Dietary Reference Intakes (DRI) published by www.nap.edu.

TABLE 9.19. DIETARY REFERENCE INTAKES (DRI) OF MINERAL SELENIUM

Age	RDA/AI*	UL
	µg/d	µg/d
Infants		
0–6 mo	15*	45
7–12 mo	20*	60
Children		
1–3 y	20	90
4–8 y	30	150
Males		
9–13 y	40	280
14 y and up	55	400
Females		
9–13 y	40	280
14 y and up	55	400
Pregnancy		
18–50 y	60	400
Lactation		
18–50 y	70	400

RDA = Recommended Daily Allowance
*AI = Adequate Intake
UL = Tolerable Upper Intake Value
ND = not determined
µg = microgram; d = day

The values are adapted and summarized from the table of the Dietary Reference Intakes (DRI) published by www.nap.edu.

TABLE 9.20. DIETARY REFERENCE INTAKES (DRI) OF MINERAL PHOSPHORUS

Age	RDA/AI*	UL
	mg/d	mg/d
Infants		
0–6 mo	100*	ND
7–12 mo	275*	ND
Children		
1–3 y	460	3,000
4–8 y	500	3,000
Males		
9–18 y	1,250	4,000
19–70 y	700	4,000
70 y and up	700	3,000
Females		
9–18 y	1,250	4,000
19–70 y	700	4,000
70 y and up	700	3,000
Pregnancy		
under 18 y	1,250	3,500
19–50 y	700	3,500
Lactation		
under 18 y	1,250	4,000
19–50 y	700	4,000

RDA = Recommended Daily Allowance
*AI = Adequate Intake
UL = Tolerable Upper Intake Value
ND = not determined
mg = milligram; d = day

The values are adapted and summarized from the table of the Dietary Reference Intakes (DRI) published by www.nap.edu.

TABLE 9.21. DIETARY REFERENCE INTAKES (DRI) OF MINERAL ZINC

Age	RDA/AI*	UL
	mg/d	mg/d
Infants		
0–6	2*	4
7–12 mo	3	5
Children		
1–3 y	3	7
4–8 y	5	12
Males		
9–13 y	8	23
14–18 y	11	34
19 y and up	11	40
Females		
9–13 y	8	23
14–18 y	9	34
19 y and up	8	40
Pregnancy		
under 18 y	12	34
19–50 y	11	40
Lactation		
under 18 y	13	34
19–50 y	12	40

RDA = Recommended Daily Allowance
*AI = Adequate Intake
UL = Tolerable Upper Intake Value
ND = not determined
mg = milligram; d = day

The values are adapted and summarized from the table of the Dietary Reference Intakes (DRI) published by www.nap.edu.

TABLE 9.22. CALORIE CONTENT
OF SELECTED FOODS

Food	Portion Size	Calories
Apple	1	80
Banana	1	100
Beans, green cooked	½ cup	18
Bread, whole wheat	1 slice	56
Butter	1 tablespoon	100
Carrot	1 medium	34
Cheese	1 ounce	107–14
Corn on the cob	5½ inches	160
Egg	1 large	80
Ice cream	½ cup	135
Kidney beans, cooked	½ cup	110
Meat	3 ounces	200–250
Milk, whole	1 cup	150
Milk, skim	1 cup	85
Orange	1	65
Peach	1	38
Peanuts	1 ounce	172
Pear	1	100
Peas	½ cup	86
Potato chips	10 chips	115
Rice, cooked	½ cup	10
Shrimp	3 ounces	78
Tuna	3 ounces	78
Yogurt, low fat	1 cup	140

From K. N. Prasad and K. C. Prasad, *Fight Cancer with Vitamins and Supplements: A Guide to Prevention and Treatment,* Rochester, Vt.: Healing Arts Press, 2001.

TABLE 9.23. FAT CONTENT
OF SELECTED FOODS

Food	Portion Size	Grams/Portion
Avocado	⅛	4
Bacon, crisp	2 slices	6
Beef, roast	3 ounces	26
Biscuit	1	4
Bread, whole wheat	1 slice	1
Cheese, cheddar	1 ounce	9
Chicken, baked, with skin	3 ounces	11
Chicken, baked, without skin	3 ounces	6
Cornbread	1 piece	7
Egg, boiled	1	6
Ice cream	½ cup	7
Margarine	1 teaspoon	4
Mayonnaise	1 tablespoon	11
Milk, whole	1 cup	8
Milk, skim	1 cup	1
Oatmeal, cooked	½ cup	1
Peanut butter	1 tablespoon	7
Pork chop	3 ounces	19
Shrimp	3 ounces	0.9
Sour cream	1 tablespoon	3
Tuna	3 ounces	0.9
Vegetable oil	1 teaspoon	5
Yogurt, low fat	1 cup	4

From K. N. Prasad and K. C. Prasad, *Fight Cancer with Vitamins and Supplements: A Guide to Prevention and Treatment,* Rochester, Vt.: Healing Arts Press, 2001.

TABLE 9.24. FIBER CONTENT
OF SELECTED FOODS

Food	Portion Size	Grams/Portion
Apple, with skin	1	3
Bread, white	1 slice	0.8
Bread, whole wheat	1 slice	1.3
Broccoli	½ cup	3.2
Carrot, raw	1 medium	2.4
Cereal, all-bran	1 cup	25.6
Cereal, raisin bran	1 cup	6
Corn	½ cup	4.6
Muffin, bran	1	4.2
Pear, with skin	1	3.8
Raspberries	½ cup	4.6

From K. N. Prasad and K. C. Prasad, *Fight Cancer with Vitamins and Supplements: A Guide to Prevention and Treatment,* Rochester, Vt.: Healing Arts Press, 2001.

CONCLUDING REMARKS

The initial nutritional guidelines, Recommended Daily Allowances (RDAs), have been replaced by Dietary Reference Intakes (DRIs) and are currently used by the United States and Canada. The DRI values of nutrients are sufficient for the growth and development of 97 to 98 percent of healthy individuals. The DRI values for carotenoids, alpha-lipoic acid, N-acetylcysteine, coenzyme Q10, and L-carnitine have not been determined; optimal values needed for prevention or improved management of cancer is not known. Therapeutic doses of antioxidants inhibit the growth of cancer cells but not of normal cells, whereas preventive doses of antioxidants do not affect the growth of cancer cells or normal cells. This distinction between the effects of therapeutic doses and preventive doses of antioxidants is often ignored when evaluating the effectiveness of these micronutrients in cancer prevention or treatment. Both preventive and therapeutic doses of micronutrients are higher than the RDA values.

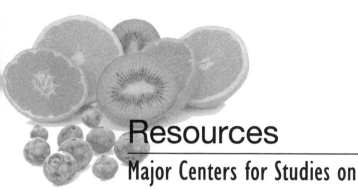

Resources

Major Centers for Studies on Antioxidants and Cancer

Adele R. Decof Cancer Center
The Roger Williams Medical Center
825 Chalkstone Avenue
Providence, Rhode Island 02908

Anderson Cancer Center
University of Texas
Scott Lippman, M.D.
1515 Holcombe Boulevard
Houston, Texas 77030

Arizona Cancer Center at UMC North
3838 N. Campbell Avenue
Tucson, Arizona 85719–1454

Arizona Cancer Center at UMC Orange Grove
1891 W. Orange Grove Road
Tucson, Arizona 85704

Beth Israel Deaconess Medical Center
Department of Surgery
Harvard Medical School

330 Brookline Avenue
Boston, Massachusetts 02215

Beverly Hills Cancer Center
8900 Wilshire Boulevard
Beverly Hills, California 90211

The Cancer Center
May Medical
615 N. Bonita Avenue
Panama City, Florida 32401

Cancer Research Center of Hawaii
University of Hawaii
1236 Lauhala Street
Honolulu, Hawaii 96913

Cancer Research Institute
Queen's University
10 Stuart Street
Kingston, Ontario K7L3N6, Canada

Cancer Therapy and Research Center
UT Health Sciences Center
South Texas Medical Center Campus

7979 Wurzbach Road
San Antonio, Texas 78229

Cancer Treatment Center of America
Midwestern Regional Medical Center
2530 Elisha Avenue
Zion, Illinois 60099

Catalan Institute of Oncology
Unit of Nutrition, Environment and
Cancer
Barcelona, Spain

**Chao Family Comprehensive Cancer
Center**
University of California at Irvine
Frank L. Meyskens Jr., M.D.
101 The City Drive, Building 23,
Route 81
Orange, California 92868

**City of Hope Comprehensive Cancer
Center**
1500 East Duarte Road
Duarte, California 91010

Dana-Farber Cancer Institute
44 Binney Street
Boston, Massachusetts 02115

The Danish Cancer Society
Institute of Cancer Epidemiology
Strandboulevarden 49
DK-2100 Copenhagen, Denmark

Duke Comprehensive Cancer Center
2424 Erwin Road
Hock Plaza, Suite 601
Durham, North Carolina 27705

Duke Oncology Network
3100 Tower Boulevard
Box 80
Durham, North Carolina 27707

European Institute of Oncology
Via Ripamonti 435
20141 Milano, Italy

**Fred Hutchinson Cancer Research
Center**
1100 Fairview Avenue N.
P.O. Box 19024
Seattle, Washington 98109

German Cancer Research Center
Division of Clinical Epidemiology
Im Neuenheimer Feld 280
D-69120 Heidelberg, Germany

Grace Cancer Drug Center
Rosewell Park Memorial Institute
Elm and Carlton Streets
Buffalo, New York 14263

**Herbert Irving Comprehensive
Cancer Center**
New York–Presbyterian Cancer Center
630 West 168 Street
New York, New York 10032

Hillman Cancer Center
UPMC Cancer Centers
515 Center Avenue
Pittsburg, Pennsylvania 15232

**Holden Comprehensive Cancer
Center**
University of Iowa
5970Z JPP
Iowa City, Iowa 53242–1002

Hotel-Dieu de Montreal Hospital
Department of Nutrition
University of Montreal
P.O. Box 6128, Station Centre-ville
Montreal, Quebec H3C3J7

Institute of Integrative Cancer Care
Keith L. Block, M.D.
1800 Sherman Avenue
Evanston, Illinois 60201

International Agency for Research
on Cancer
Unit of Nutrition and Cancer
150 Cours Albert-Thomas, 69372
Lyon Cedex 08, France

ISPO—Cancer Research and
Prevention Institute
Molecular and Nutritional
Epidemiology Unit
Via Cosimo il Vecchio 2
50139 Florence, Italy

King Hussein Cancer Center
Queen Rania Al Abdullah Street
P.O. Box 1269
Amman 11941
Hashemite Kingdom of Jordan

The Lacks Cancer Center
Saint Mary's Hospital
250 Cherry Street
Grand Rapids, Michigan 49503

Linus Pauling Institute
Oregon State University
Balz Frei, Ph.D.
571Weniger Hall
Corvallis, Oregon 97331–6512

Masonic Cancer Center
University of Minnesota
Mayo Mail Code 806
420 Delware Street SE
Minneapolis, Minnesota 55455

Memorial Sloan-Kettering Cancer
Center
1275 York Avenue
New York, New York 10065

Moffitt Cancer Center
12902 Magnolia Drive
Tampa, Florida 33612

MRC Center for Nutritional
Epidemiology and Cancer
Prevention and Survival
Department of Public Health and
Primary Care
University of Cambridge
Trinity Lane
Cambridge, CB18RN, UK

National Cancer Institute of Canada
Cancer Clinical Trial Division
Cancer Research Institute
Queen's University
10 Stuart Street, Suite 300
Kingston, ON K73N6, Canada

National Institutes of Health
Nutritional Science Research Group
Division of Cancer Prevention
National Cancer Institute
Clinical Center, Department of
Nutrition
6130 Executive Boulevard
Rockville, Maryland 20892

Norris Cotton Cancer Center
Dartmouth-Hitchcock Medical Center
One Medical Center Drive
Lebanon, New Hampshire 03756

Nutrition and Cancer Center
Marshall University
Robert C. Byrd Biotechnology Science
Center
1700 Third Avenue
Huntington, West Virginia 25703

**Nutrition at Weymouth-
Commonwealth Atrius Cancer
Center**
51 Performance Drive
Weymouth, Massachusetts 02189

Premier Micronutrient Corporation
Antioxidant Research Institute
14 Galli Drive
Novato, California 94949

**The Prostatitis and Prostate Cancer
Center**
Diagnostic Center for Disease
1250 South Tamiami Trail, Suite 101
Sarasota, Florida 34239

**The S. Daniel International Center
for Health and Nutrition**
Ben-Gurion University of Negev
Hatmarim Boulevard
Eilat, 88000
Israel

**Simms/Mann-UCLA Center for
Integrative Oncology**
200 UCLA Medical Plaza, Suite 502
Los Angeles, California 90095–6934

Simone Protective Cancer Center
Charles Simone, M.D.
123 Franklin Corner Road
Lawrenceville, New Jersey 08648

Siteman Cancer Center
Washington University School of
Medicine
660 S. Euclid
Box 8100
St. Louis, Missouri 63110

Stanford Cancer Center
Nutrition and Metabolism Laboratory
Stanford Center for Integrative
Medicine
875 Blake Wilbur Drive
Stanford, California 94305

Sutter Cancer Center
2801 L Street
Sacramento, California 95816

UAB Comprehensive Cancer Center
University of Alabama
18 Street
Birmingham, Alabama 35294

**UCLA Johnson Comprehensive
Cancer Center**
8-684 Factor Building, Box 951781
Los Angeles, California 90095–1781

UCSD Moores Cancer Center
9500 Gilman Drive, M/C 0176T
La Jolla, California 92093–0176

**UNC Lineberger Comprehensive
Cancer Center**
University of North Carolina
101 Manning Drive
Chapel Hill, North Carolina 27514

**University of Cologne Medical
Center**
Professor Josef Beuth, M.D.
Joseph-Stelzmann-strabe-9
Building 35a
50931 Cologne, Germany

University of Kansas Medical Center
Jeanne Drisko, M.D., C.N.S., F.A.C.N.
Riordan Endowed Professor of
Orthomolecular Medicine
Director, Program in Integrative
Medicine Complementary and
Alternative Therapies
3901 Rainbow Blvd.
Kansas City, Kansas 66160

**University of Pennsylvania
Medical School**
Department of Radiation Oncology
Ann R. Kennedy, Ph.D.
3600 Market Street
Philadelphia, Pennsylvania 19104

**University of Colorado Cancer
Center**
1665 Aurora Court
Aurora, Colorado 80045

**University of Michigan
Comprehensive Cancer Center**
1500 East Medical Center Drive
Ann Arbor, Michigan 48109

University of Oxford Cancer
Epidemiology Unit
Roosevelt Drive
University of Oxford
Oxford, OX37XP, UK

University of Virginia Cancer Center
1222 Jefferson Park Avenue
P.O. Box 800334
Charlottesville, Virginia 22908

**USDA Human Nutrition Research
Center for Aging**
Tufts University
711 Washington Street
Boston, Massachusetts 02111

VCU Massey Cancer Center
401 College Street
P.O. Box 980037
Richmond, Virginia 23198–0037

Virtua Fox Chase Cancer Program
175 Madison Avenue
Mount Holly, New Jersey 08060

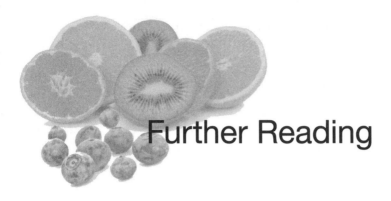

Further Reading

Abdel-Rassoul, G., et al. "Neurobehavioral Effects Among Inhabitants Around Mobile Phone Base Stations." *Neurotoxicology* 28 (2) (2007): 434–40.

Adlercreutz, H., et al. "Estrogen Metabolism and Excretion in Oriental and Caucasian Women." J. Natl. Cancer Inst. 86 (1994): 1643–45.

Aerts, I. et al. "Retinoblastoma. Orphanet." *J Rare Dis* 1 (2006): 31.

Ahern, T. P., et al. "Lifetime Tobacco Smoke Exposure and Breast Cancer Incidence." *Cancer Causes Control* (2009).

Albanes, D., et al. "Effects of Alpha-tocopherol and Beta-carotene Supplements on Cancer Incidence in the Alpha-Tocopherol Beta-Carotene Cancer Prevention Study." *American Journal of Clinical Nutrition* 62 (1995): 1427S–1430S.

Alberts, D. S., et al. "Lack of Effect of a High-Fiber Cereal Supplement on the Recurrence of Colorectal Adenomas. Phoenix Colon Cancer Prevention Physicians' Network." *New England of Journal of Medicine* 342 (2000): 1156–62.

Alkhenizan, A., and K. Hafez. "The Role of Vitamin E in the Prevention of Cancer: A Meta-Analysis of Randomized Controlled Trials." *Annals of Saudi Medicine* 27 (2007): 409–14.

The Alpha-tocopherol Beta-carotene Cancer Prevention Study Group. "The Effect of Vitamin E and Beta-carotene on the Incidence of Lung and Other Cancers in Male Smokers." *New England Journal of Medicine* 330 (1994): 1029–35.

Ames, B. N., "Dietary Carcinogens and Anticarcinogens. Oxygen Radicals and Degenerative Diseases." *Science* 221 (1983): 1256–64.

Amis, E. S., et.al. "American College of Radiology White Paper on Radiation Dose in Medicine." *J Am Coll Radiol* 4 (5) (2007): 272–84.

Anderson, K. E., et al. "Nutrient Regulation of Chemical Metabolism in Humans." *Federation Proceedings* 44 (1985): 130–33.

Argyriou, A. A., et al. "A Randomized Controlled Trial Evaluating the Efficacy and Safety of Vitamin E Supplementation for Protection against Cisplatin-Induced Peripheral Neuropathy: Final Results." *Supportive Care in Cancer* 14 (2006): 1134–40.

Argyriou, A. A., et al. "Vitamin E for Prophylaxis against Chemotherapy-Induced

Neuropathy: A Randomized Controlled Trial." *Neurology* 64 (2005): 26–31.

Babu, J. R., et al. "Salubrious Effect of Vitamin C and Vitamin E on Tamoxifen- treated Women in Breast Cancer with Reference to Plasma Lipid and Lipoprotein Levels." *Cancer lett* 151 (2000): 1–5.

Bairati, I., et al. "Randomized Trial of Antioxidant Vitamins to Prevent Acute Adverse Effects of Radiation Therapy in Head and Neck Cancer Patients." *Journal of Clinical Oncology* 23 (2005): 5805–13.

Balansky, R. M., et al. "Effects of N-acetylcysteine in an Esophageal Carcinogenesis Model in Rats Treated with Diethylnitrosamine and Diethyldithiocarbamate." *International Journal of Cancer* 98 (2002): 493–97.

Band, P. R., et al. "Cohort Study of Air Canada Pilots: Mortality, Cancer Incidence, and Leukemia Risk." *Am J Epidemiol* 143 (2) (1996): 137–43.

BEIR VII, Phase 2. Washington, D.C.: The National Academies Press, 2006.

Ben-Amotz, A., et al. "Effect of Natural Beta-carotene Supplementation in Children Exposed to Radiation from the Chernobyl Accident." *Radiat Environ Biophys* 37 (3) (1998): 187–93.

Benner, S. E., et al. "Regression of Oral Leukoplakia with Alpha-tocopherol: A Community Clinical Oncology Program Chemoprevention Study." *Journal of the National Cancer Institute* 85 (1993): 44–47.

Beresford, S. A., et al. "Low-Fat Dietary Pattern and Risk of Colorectal Cancer: The Women's Health Initiative Randomized Controlled Dietary Modification Trial." *JAMA* 295 (2006): 643–54.

Berkson, B. M., D. M. Rubin, and A. J. Berkson. "The Long-Term Survival of a Patient with Pancreatic Cancer with Metastases to the Liver after Treatment with the Intravenous Alpha-Lipoic Acid/Low-Dose Naltrexone Protocol." *Integrative Cancer Therapies* 5 (2006): 83–89.

Berrington de Gonzalez, A., and S. Darby. "Risk of Cancer from Diagnostic X-rays: Estimates for the UK and 14 Other Countries." *Lancet* 363 (9406) (2004): 345–51.

Biasco, G., and G. M. Paganelli. "European Trials on Dietary Supplementation for Cancer Prevention." *Annals of the New York Academy of Sciences* 889 (1999): 152–56.

Blot, W. J., et al. "Nutrition Intervention Trials in Linxian, China: Supplementation with Specific Vitamin/Mineral Combinations, Cancer Incidence, and Disease-Specific Mortality in the General Population." *Journal of the National Cancer Institute* 85 (1993): 1483–92.

Blumenthal, R. D., et al. "Anti-oxidant Vitamins Reduce Normal Tissue Toxicity Induced by Radio-immunotherapy." *Int J Cancer* 86 (2) (2000): 276–80.

Borek, C., et al. "Ozone Acts Alone and Synergistically with Ionizing Radiation to Induce In Vitro Neoplastic Transformation." *Carcinogenesis* 7 (9) (1986): 1611–13.

Boutwell, R. "Biology and Biochemistry of Two-steps Carcinogenesis." In *Modulation and Mediation of Cancer by Vitamins*. Basel: Karger, 1983.

Brenner, D. J., and R. K. Sachs. "Estimating Radiation-induced Cancer Risks at Very

Low Doses: Rationale for Using a Linear No-threshold Approach." *Radiat Environ Biophys* 44 (4) (2006): 253–56.

Brenner, D., et al. "Estimated Risks of Radiation-induced Fatal Cancer from Pediatric CT." *AJR Am J Roentgenol* 176 (2) (2001): 289–96.

Briviba, K., et al. "Beta-carotene Inhibits Growth of Human Colon Carcinoma Cells In Vitro by Induction of Apoptosis." *Biological Chemistry* 382 (2001): 1663–68.

Buja, A., et al. "Cancer Incidence Among Male Military and Civil Pilots and Flight Attendants: An Analysis on Published Data." *Toxicol Ind Health* 21 (10) (2005): 273–82.

Buring, J., and C. H. Hennekens. "Antioxidant Vitamins in Cancer: The Physician's Health Study and Women's Health Study." In *Nutrients in Cancer Prevention and Treatment*, by K. N. Prasad, L. Santamaria, and R. M. Williams, 223. Totowa, N.J.: Humana Press, 1995.

Cameron, E., L. Pauling, and B. Leibowitz. "Ascorbic Acid and Cancer. A review." *Cancer Research* 39 (1979): 663–81.

Cascinu, S., et al. "Neuroprotective Effect of Reduced Glutathione on Oxaliplatin-Based Chemotherapy in Advanced Colorectal Cancer: A Randomized, Double-Blind, Placebo-Controlled Trial." *Journal of Clinical Oncology* 20 (2002): 3478–83.

Cerqueira, E. M., et al. "Genotoxic Effects of X-rays on Keratinized Mucosa Cells During Paroramic Dental Radiography." *Dentomaxillofac Radiol* (37) (2008): 398–403.

Chen, C. S., J. A. Squire, and P. G. Wells. "Reduced Tumorigenesis in p53 Knockout Mice Exposed In Utero to Low-Dose Vitamin E." *Cancer* 115 (2009): 1563–75.

Chen, Q., et al. "Ascorbate in Pharmacologic Concentrations Selectively Generates Ascorbate Radical and Hydrogen Peroxide in Extracellular Fluid In Vivo." *Proceedings of the National Academy of Science of the United States of America* 104 (2007): 8749–54.

Chen, Q., et al. "Pharmacologic Ascorbic Acid Concentrations Selectively Kill Cancer Cells: Action as a Pro-Drug to Deliver Hydrogen Peroxide to Tissues." *Proceedings of the National Academy of Sciences of the United States of America* 102 (2005): 13604–9.

Chlebowski, R. T., et al. "Calcium Plus Vitamin D Supplementation and the Risk of Breast Cancer." *Journal of the National Cancer Institute* 100 (2008): 1581–91.

Chocolatewala, N. M., and P. Chaturvedi. "Role of Human Papilloma Virus in the Oral Carcinogenesis: An Indian Perspective." *J Cancer Res Ther* 5 (2) (2009): 71–77.

Chodick, G., et al. "Excess Lifetime Cancer Mortality Risk Attributable to Radiation Exposure from Computed Tomography Examinations in Children." *Isr Med Assoc J* 9 (8) (2007): 584–87.

Cohen, M., and H. N. Bhagavan. "Ascorbic Acid and Gastrointestinal Cancer." *Journal of the American College of Nutrition* 14 (1995): 565–78.

Cole, B. F., et al. "Folic Acid for the Prevention of Colorectal Adenomas: A Randomized Clinical Trial." *JAMA* 297 (2007): 2351–59.

Conney, A. H., et al. "Inhibitory Effect of Curcumin and Some Related Dietary

Compounds on Tumor Promotion and Arachidonic Acid Metabolism in Mouse Skin." *Advances in Enzyme Regulation* 31 (1991): 385–96.

Cotran, R. S., V. Kumar., and T. Collins. "Disease of Immunity." *Pathologic Basis of Disease,* 188–259. New York: W. B. Saunders Company, 1999.

Coulter, I. D., et al. "Antioxidants Vitamin C and Vitamin E for the Prevention and Treatment of Cancer." *Journal of General Internal Medicine* 21 (2006): 735–44.

Creagan, E. T., C. G. Moerrtel, and J. R. O'Fallon. "Failure of High-Dose Vitamin C (Ascorbic Acid) Therapy to Benefit Patients with Advanced Cancer." *New England Journal of Medicine* 301 (1979): 687–90.

Crous-Bou, M., et al. "Lifetime History of Alcohol Consumption and K-ras Mutations in Pancreatic Ductal Adenocarcinoma." *Environ Mol Mutagen* 50 (5) (2009): 421–30.

Crowe, D. L., R. Kim, and R. A. Chandraratna. "Retinoic Acid Differentially Regulates Cancer Cell Proliferation via Dose-Dependent Modulation of the Mitogen-Activated Protein Kinase Pathway." *Molecular Cancer Research* 1 (2003): 532–40.

Dagenais, G. R., et al. "Impact of Cigarette Smoking in High-Risk Patients Participating in a Clinical Trial. A Substudy from the Heart Outcomes Prevention Evaluation (HOPE) Trial." *European Journal of Cardiovascular Prevention and Rehabilitation* 12 (2005): 75–81.

DeCosse, J. J., H. H. Miller, and M. L. Lesser. "Effect of Wheat Fiber and Vitamins C and E on Rectal Polyps in Patients with Familial Adenomatous Polyposis." *Journal of the National Cancer Institute* 81 (1989): 1290–97.

De Flora, S., G. A. Rossi, and A. De Flora. "Metabolic, Desmutagenic and Anticarcinogenic Effects of N-acetylcysteine." *Respiration* 50 Suppl 1 (1986): 43–49.

Dennert, G., and M. Horneber. "Selenium for Alleviating the Side Effects of Chemotherapy, Radiotherapy and Surgery in Cancer Patients." *Cochrane Database of Systematic Reviews* 3 (2006): CD005037.

Ding, E. L., et al. "Interaction of Estrogen Therapy with Calcium and Vitamin D Supplementation on Colorectal Cancer Risk: Reanalysis of Women's Health Initiative Randomized Trial." *International Journal of Cancer* 122 (2008): 1690–94.

Dion, P. W., et al. "The Effect of Dietary Ascorbic Acid and Alpha-tocopherol on Fecal Mutagenicity." *Mutation Research* 102 (1982): 27–37.

DiPaolo, J. A., and P. J. Donovan. "In Vitro Morphologic Transformation of Syrian Hamster Cells by U.V.-irradiation is Enhanced by X-irridation and Unaffected by Chemical Carcinogens." *Int J Radiat Biol Relat Stud Phys Chem Med* 30 (1) (1976): 41–53.

DiPaolo, J. A., et al. "Cellular and Molecular Alterations in Human Epithelial Cells Transformed by Recombinant Human Papillomavirus DNA." *Crit Rev Oncog* 4 (4) (1993): 337–60.

DiPaolo, J. A., P. J. Donavan, and N. C. Popewscu. "Kinetecs of Syrian Hamster Cells During X-irradiation Enhancement of Transformation *In Vitro* by Chemical Carcinogen." *Radiation Res* 66 (1976): 310.

Drisko, J. A., J. Chapman, and V. J. Hunter. "The Use of Antioxidants with First-Line

Chemotherapy in Two Cases of Ovarian Cancer." *Journal of the American College of Nutrition* 22 (2003): 118–23.

Duan, L., et al. "Passive Smokig and Risk of Oesophageal and Gastric Adenocarcinomas." *Br J Cancer* 100 (9) (2009): 1483–85.

Duthie, G. G., J. R. Arthur, and W. P. James. "Effects of Smoking and Vitamin E on Blood Antioxidant Status." *American Journal of Clinical Nutrition* 53 (1991): 1061S–1063S.

Duthie, S. J., et al. "Antioxidant Supplementation Decreases Oxidative DNA Damage in Human Lymphocytes." *Cancer Research* 56 (1996): 1291–95.

El-Habit, O. H., et al. "The Modifying Effect of Beta-carotene on Gamma Radiation-induced Eelevation of Oxidative Reactions and Genotoxicity in Male Rats." *Mutat Res* 466 (2) (2000): 179–86.

Ellinger, S., et al. "Tomatoes and Lycopene in Prevention and Therapy—Is There any Evidence for Prostate Diseases?" *Aktuelle Urologie* 40 (2009): 37–43.

Ershoff, B. H., and C. W. Steers Jr. "Antioxidants and Survival Time of Mice Exposed to Mutliple Sublethal Doses of X-irradiation." *Proc Soc Exp Biol Med* 104 (1960): 274–76.

Franceschi, S., et al. "Human Papillomavirus and Cancers of the Upper Aerodigestive Tract: A Review of Epidemiological and Experimental Evidence." *Cancer Epidemiol Biomarkers Prev* 5 (7) (1996): 567–75.

Fraser, G. E. "Associations between diet and cancer, ischemic heart disease, and all-cause mortality in non-hispanic white California Seventh-Day Adventists." *Am J Clin Nutr* 70 (1999): 532S–538S.

Fukushima, S., et al. "L-ascorbic Acid Amplification of Second-Stage Bladder Carcinogenesis Promotion by NaHCO3." *Cancer Research* 48 (1988): 6317–20.

Gallicchio, L., et al. "Carotenoids and the Risk of Developing Lung Cancer: A Systematic Review." *American Journal of Clinical Nutrition* 88 (2008): 372–83.

Ganmaa, D., et al. "Coffee, Tea, Caffeine and Risk of Breast Cancer: A 22-year Follow-up." *Int J Cancer* 122 (9) (2008): 2071–76.

Garewal, H. "Beta-carotene and Antioxidant Nutrients in Oral Cancer Prevention." In *Nutrients in Cancer Prevention and Treatment* by K. N. Prasad, R. M. Williams, 235–47. Totawa, N.J.: Humana Press, 1995.

Gaziev, A. I., et al. "Dietary Supplements of Antioxidants Reduce HPRT Mutant Frequency in Slenocytes of Aging Mice." *Mutat Res* 338 (1–6) (1995): 77–86.

Genkinger, J. M., et al. "Alcohol Intake and Pancreatic Cancer Risk: A Pooled Analysis of Fourteen Cohort Studies." *Cancer Epidemiol Biomarkers Prev* 18 (3) (2009): 765–76.

Gerss, J., and W. Kopcke. "The Questionable Association of Vitamin E Supplementation and Mortality—Inconsistent Results of Different Meta-Analytic Approaches." *Cellular and Molecular Biology* 55 Suppl, OL (2009): 1111–20.

Giovannucci, E., et al. *Cancer Res* 54 (1994): 2390.

Gonzalez, M. J., et al. "Orthomolecular Oncology Review: Ascorbic Acid and Cancer 25 Years Later." *Integrative Cancer Therapies* 4 (2005): 32–44.

Gorham, E. D., et al. "Optimal Vitamin D Status for Colorectal Cancer Prevention: A Quantitative Meta Analysis." *American Journal of Preventive Medicine* 32 (2007): 210–16.

Gorham, E. D., et al. "Vitamin D and Prevention of Colorectal Cancer." *Journal of Steroid Biochemistry and Molecular Biology* 97 (2005): 179–94.

Grau, M. V., et al. "Vitamin D, Calcium Supplementation, and Colorectal Adenomas: Results of a Randomized Trial." *Journal of the National Cancer Institute* 95 (2003): 1765–71.

Greenberg, E. R., et al. "A Clinical Trial of Antioxidant Vitamins to Prevent Colorectal Adenoma. Polyp Prevention Study Group." *New England Journal of Medicine* 331 (1994): 141–47.

Guan, J., et al. "Effects of Dietary Supplements on Space Radiation-induced Oxidative Stress in Sprague-Dawley Rats." *Radiat Res* 162 (5) (2004): 572–79.

Hall, E. J. "Lessons We Have Learned from Our Children: Cancer Risks from Diagnostic Radiology." *Pediatr Radiol* 32 (10) (2002): 700–706.

Hall, E. J., and A. J. Giaccia. *Radiobiology for the Radiologist.* Philadelphia: Lippincott, Williams & Wilkins, 2006.

Han, Y. Y., et al. "Cell Phone Use and Acoustic Neuroma: The Need for Standardized Questionnaires and Access to Industry Data." *Surg Neurol* (2009).

Hao, J., et al. "Effect of Alpha-tocopherol, N-acetylcysteine and Omeprazole on Esophageal Adenocarcinoma Formation in a Rat Surgical Model." *International Journal of Cancer* 124 (2009): 1270–75.

Harapanhalli, R. S., et al. "Antioxidant Effects of Vitamin C in Mice Following X-irradiation." *Res Commun Mol Pathol Pharmacol* 94 (3) (1996): 271–87.

Hardell, L., and C. Sage. "Biological Effects from Electromagnetic Field Exposure and Public Exposure Standards." *Biomed Pharmacother* 62 (2) (2008): 104–9.

Harnack, L., et al. "Relationship of Folate, Vitamin B6, vitamin B12, and Methionine Intake to Incidence of Colorectal Cancers." *Nutrition and Cancer* 43 (2002): 152–58.

Hayatsu, H., T. Hayatsu, and Y. Wataya. "Use of Blue Cotton for Detection of Mutagenicity in Human Feces Excreted After Ingestion of Cooked Meat." *Environ Health Perspect* 67 (1986): 31–34.

Heaney, M. L., et al. "Vitamin C Antagonizes the Cytotoxic Effects of Antineoplastic Drugs." *Cancer Research* 68 (2008): 8031–38.

Hemelt, M., et al. "The Effect of Smoking on the Male Excess of Bladder Cancer: A Meta-analysis and Geographical Analyses." *Int J Cancer* 124 (2) (2009): 412–19.

Hennekens, C. H. "Antioxidant Vitamins and Cancer." *American Journal of Medicine* 97 (1994): 2S–4S; discussion 22S–28S.

Hennekens, C. H., et al. "Lack of Effect of Long-Term Supplementation with Beta-carotene on the Incidence of Malignant Neoplasms and Cardiovascular Disease." *New England Journal of Medicine* 334 (1996): 1145–49.

Hernandez J., et al. "The Modulation of Prostate Cancer Risk with Alpha-tocopherol:

A Pilot Randomized, Controlled Clinical Trial." *Journal of Urology* 174 (2005): 519–22.

Hill, D. L., C. J. Grubbs. "Retinoids as Chemopreventive and Anticancer Agents in Intact Animals (Review)." *Anticancer Research* 2 (1982): 111–24.

Ho, Y. S., et al. "Dihydrolipoic Acid Inhibits Skin Tumor Promotion through Anti-Inflammation and Anti-Oxidation." *Biochemical Pharmacology* 73 (2007): 1786–95.

Hoenjet, K. M., et al. "Effect of a Nutritional Supplement Containing Vitamin E, Selenium, Vitamin C and Coenzyme Q10 on Serum PSA in Patients with Hormonally Untreated Carcinoma of the Prostate: A Randomised Placebo-Controlled Study." *European Urology* 47 (2005): 433–39.

Hogervorst, J. G., et al. "Lung Cancer Risk in Relation to Dietary Acrylamide Intake." *J Natl Cancer Inst* 101 (9) (2009): 651–62.

Homann, N., et al. "Alcohol and Colorectal Cancer: The Role of Alcohol Dehydrogenase 1C Polymorphism." *Alcohol Clin Exp Res* 33 (3) (2009): 551–56.

Hong, S. W., et al. "Ascorbate (Vitamin C) Induces Cell Death through the Apoptosis-Inducing Factor in Human Breast Cancer Cells." *Oncology Reports* 18 (2007): 811–15.

Hwang, E. S., and P. E. Bowen. "Cell Cycle Arrest and Induction of Apoptosis by Lycopene in LNCaP Human Prostate Cancer Cells." *Journal of Medicinal Food* 7 (2004): 284–89.

Ishihara, J., et al. "Low Intake of Vitamin B6 Is Associated with Increased Risk of Colorectal Cancer in Japanese Men." *Journal of Nutrition* 137 (2007): 1808–14.

Ishitani, K., et al. "Caffeine Consumption and the Risk of Breast Cancer in a Large Prospective Cohort of Women." *Arch Intern Med* 168 (18) (2008): 2022–31.

Jaakkola, K., et al. "Treatment with Antioxidant and Other Nutrients in Combination with Chemotherapy and Irradiation in Patients with Small-Cell Lung Cancer." *Anticancer Research* 12 (1992): 599–606.

Jaszewski, R., et al. "Folic Acid Supplementation Inhibits Recurrence of Colorectal Adenomas: A Randomized Chemoprevention Trial." *World Journal of Gastroenterology* 14 (2008): 4492–98.

Jedrychowski, W., and U. Maugeri. "An Apple a Day May Hold Colorectal Cancer at Bay: Recent Evidence from a Case-Control Study." *Reviews on Environmental Health* 24 (2009): 59–74.

Johnson, K. C. "Accumulating Evidence on Passive and Active Smoking and Breast Cancer Risk." *Int J Cancer* 117 (4) (2005): 619–28.

Johnson, K. C., J. Hu, and Y. Mao. "Passive and Active Smoking and Breast Cancer Risk in Canada, 1994–97." *Cancer Causes Control* 11 (3) (2000): 211–21.

Judy, W. V., K. Folkers, and J. Hall. "Improved Long-Term Survival in Coenzyme Q10 Treated Congestive Heart Failure Patients Compared to Conventionally Treated Patients." In *Biomedical and Clincial Aspects of Coenzyme Q,* edited by K. Folkers, G. P. Littarro, and T. Yamagami, 291–98. Amsterdam: Elsevier, 1991.

Kabat, G. C., et al. "Longitudinal Study of Serum Carotenoid, Retinol, and Tocopherol Concentrations in Relation to Breast Cancer Risk among Postmenopausal Women." *American Journal of Clinical Nutrition* 90 (2009): 162–69.

Kan, P., et al. "Cellular Phone Use and Brain Tumor: A Meta-analysis." *J Neurooncol* 86 (1) (2008): 71–78.

Kant, A. K., et al. "A Prospective Study of Diet Quality and Mortality in Women." *JAMA* 283 (2000): 2109–15.

Kennedy, A. R., and N. I. Krinsky. "Effects of Retinoids, Beta-carotene, and Canthaxanthin on UV- and X-ray-induced Transformation of C3H10T1/2 Cells In Vitro." *Nutr Cancer* 22 (3) (1994): 219–32.

Kennedy, A. R., et al. "Protection Against Adverse Biological Effects Induced by Space Radiation by the Bowman-Birk Inhibitor and Antioxidants." *Radiat Res* 166 (2) (2006): 327–32.

Kim, J. Y., et al. "In Vitro Assessment of Clastogenicity of Mobile-phone Radiation (835 MHz) Using the Alkaline Comet Assay and Chromosomal Aberration Test." *Environ Toxicol* 23 (3) (2008): 319–27.

Kirsh, V. A., et al. "Supplemental and Dietary Vitamin E, Beta-carotene, and Vitamin C Intakes and Prostate Cancer Risk." *Journal of the National Cancer Institute* 98 (2006): 245–54.

Kiyosawa, H., et al. "Cigarette Smoking Induces Formation of 8-hydroxydeoxyguanosine, One of the Oxidative DNA Damages in Human Peripheral Leukocytes." *Free Radical Research Communications* 11 (1990): 23–27.

Konopacka, M., M. Widel, and J. Rzeszowska-Wolny. "Modifying Effect of Vitamins C, E, and Beta-carotene Against Gamma-ray-induced DNA Damage in Mouse Cells." *Mutat Res* 417 (2–3) (1998): 85–94.

Korkina, L. G., I. B. Afanas'ef, and A. T. Diplock. "Antioxidant Therapy in Children Affected by Irradiation from the Chernobyl Nuclear Accident." *Biochem Soc Trans* 21 (Pt 3) (3) (1993): 314S.

Koushik, A., et al. "Fruits and Vegetables and Ovarian Cancer Risk in a Pooled Analysis of 12 Cohort Studies." *Cancer Epidemiology, Biomarkers and Prevention* 14 (2005): 2160–67.

Krinsky, N. I., "Antioxidant Functions of Carotenoids." *Free Radical Biology and Medicine* 7 (1989): 617–35.

Kristal, A. R., et al. "Dietary Patterns, Supplement Use, and the Risk of Symptomatic Benign Prostatic Hyperplasia: Results from the Prostate Cancer Prevention Trial." *American Journal of Epidemiology* 167 (2008): 925–34.

Kropp, S., and J. Chang-Claude. "Active and Passive Smoking and Risk of Breast Cancer by Age 50 Years Among German Women." *Am J Epidemiol* 156 (7) (2002): 616–26.

Kumar, B., et al. "D-alpha-tocopheryl succinate (vitamin E) Enhances Radiation-induced Chromosomal Damage Levels in Human Cancer Cells, But Reduces It in Normal Cells." *J Am Coll Nutr* 21 (4) (2002): 339–43.

Kune, G., and L. Watson. "Colorectal Cancer Protective Effects and the Dietary Micronutrients Folate, Methionine, Vitamins B₆, B₁₂, C, E, Selenium, and Lycopene." *Nutrition and Cancer* 56 (2006): 11–21.

Kurahashi, N., et al. "Coffee, Green Tea, and Caffeine Consumption and Subsequent Risk of Bladder Cancer in Relation to Smoking Status: A Prospective Study in Japan." *Cancer Sci* (2008).

Labriola, D., and R. Livingston. "Possible Interactions Between Dietary Antioxidants and Chemotherapy." *Oncology* 13 (1999): 1003–8, discussion 1008, 1011–12.

Lajous, M., et al. "Folate, Vitamin B(6), and Vitamin B(12) Intake and the Risk of Breast Cancer among Mexican Women." *Cancer Epidemiology, Biomarkers and Prevention* 15 (2006): 443–48.

Lamm, D. L., et al. "Megadose Vitamins in Bladder Cancer: A Double-Blind Clinical Trial." *Journal of Urology* 151 (1994): 21–26.

Lamson, D. W., and M. S. Brignall. "Antioxidants in Cancer Therapy; Their Actions and Interactions with Oncologic Therapies." *Alternative Medicine Review* 4 (1999): 304–29.

Langsjoen, P. H., P. H. Langsjoen, and K. Folkers. "Long-Term Efficacy and Safety of Coenzyme Q10 Therapy for Idiopathic Dilated Cardiomyopathy." *American Journal of Cardiology* 65 (1990): 521–23.

La Rosa, F. G., et al. "Inhibition of Proliferation and Expression of T-antigen in SV40 Large T-antigen Gene-induced Immortalized Cells Following Transplantations." *Cancer Lett* 113 (1–2) (1997): 55–60.

Larsson, S. C., and A. Wolk. "Coffee Consumption and Risk of Liver Cancer: A Meta-analysis." *Gastroenterology* 132 (5) (2007): 1740–45.

Lee, S. K., et al. "Vitamin C Suppresses Proliferation of the Human Melanoma Cell SK-MEL-2 through the Inhibition of Cyclooxygenase-2 (COX-2) Expression and the Modulation of Insulin-like Growth Factor II (IGF-II) Production." *Journal of Cellular Physiology* 216 (2008): 180–88.

Lin, J., et al. "Vitamins C and E and Beta-carotene Supplementation and Cancer Risk: A Randomized Controlled Trial." *Journal of the National Cancer Institute* 101 (2009): 4–23.

Lin, P. C., et al. "N-acetylcysteine Has Neuroprotective Effects against Oxaliplatin-Based Adjuvant Chemotherapy in Colon Cancer Patients: Preliminary Data." *Supportive Care in Cancer* 14 (2006): 484–87.

Lippman, S. M., et al. "Effect of Selenium and Vitamin E on Risk of Prostate Cancer and Other Cancers: The Selenium and Vitamin E Cancer Prevention Trial (SELECT)." *JAMA* 301 (2009): 39–51.

Lippman, S. M., et al. "13-cis-retinoic Acid Plus Interferon Alpha-2a: Highly Active Systemic Therapy for Squamous Cell Carcinoma of the Cervix." *Journal of the National Cancer Institute* 84 (1992): 241–45.

Lockwood, K., et al. "Apparent Partial Remission of Breast Cancer in 'High Risk' Patients Supplemented with Nutritional Antioxidants, Essential Fatty Acids and Coenzyme Q10." *Molecular Aspects of Medicine* 15 Suppl (1994): s231–40.

Lockwood, K., et al. "Progress on Therapy of Breast Cancer with Vitamin Q10 and the Regression of Metastases." *Biochemical and Biophysical Research Communications* 212 (1995): 172–77.

Logan, R. F., et al. "Aspirin and Folic Acid for the Prevention of Recurrent Colorectal Adenomas." *Gastroenterology* 134 (2008): 29–38.

Lonn, E., et al. "Effects of Long-Term Vitamin E Supplementation on Cardiovascular Events and Cancer: A Randomized Controlled Trial." *JAMA* 293 (2005): 1338–47.

Lonn, E., et al. "Effects of Ramipril and Vitamin E on Atherosclerosis: The Study to Evaluate Carotid Ultrasound Changes in Patients Treated with Ramipril and Vitamin E (SECURE)." *Circulation* 103 (2001): 919–25.

Lonn, E., et al. "Effects of Vitamin E on Cardiovascular and Microvascular Outcomes in High-Risk Patients with Diabetes: Results of the HOPE Study and MICRO-HOPE Substudy." *Diabetes Care* 25 (2002): 1919–27.

Lubet, R. A., et al. "Chemopreventive Efficacy of Anethole Trithione, N-acetyl-L-cysteine, Miconazole and Phenethylisothiocyanate in the DMBA-Induced Rat Mammary Cancer Model." *International Journal of Cancer* 72 (1997): 95–101.

Lueth, N. A., et al. "Coffee and Caffeine Intake and the Risk of Ovarian Cancer: The Iowa Women's Health Study." *Cancer Causes Control* 19 (10) (2008): 1365–72.

Ma, E., et al. "Dietary Intake of Folate, Vitamin B_6, and Vitamin B_{12}, Genetic Polymorphism of Related Enzymes, and Risk of Breast Cancer: A Case-Control Study in Brazilian Women." *BMC Cancer* 9 (2009): 122.

Malmberg, K. J., et al. "A Short-Term Dietary Supplementation of High Doses of Vitamin E Increases T Helper 1 Cytokine Production in Patients with Advanced Colorectal Cancer." *Clinical Cancer Research* 8 (2002): 1772–78.

Mann, J. F., et al. "Effects of Vitamin E on Cardiovascular Outcomes in People with Mild-to-Moderate Renal Insufficiency: Results of the HOPE Study." *Kidney International* 65 (2004): 1375–80.

Martin, K. R., et al. "Dietary N-acetyl-L-cysteine Modulates Benzo[a]pyrene-Induced Skin Tumors in Cancer-Prone p53 Haploinsufficient Tg.AC (v-Ha-ras) Mice." *Carcinogenesis* 22 (2001): 1373–78.

Martinez, M. E., et al. "Calcium, Vitamin D, and Risk of Adenoma Recurrence (United States)." *Cancer Causes and Control* 13 (2002): 213–20.

McCullough, M. J., and C. S. Farah. "The Role of Alcohol in Oral Carcinogenesis with Particular Reference to Alcohol-containing Mouthwashes." *Aust Dent J* 53 (4) (2008): 302–5.

McCullough, M. L., et al. "Dairy, Calcium, and Vitamin D Intake and Postmenopausal Breast Cancer Risk in the Cancer Prevention Study II Nutrition Cohort." *Cancer Epidemiology, Biomarkers and Prevention* 14 (2005): 2898–904.

McKeown-Eyssen, G., et al. "A Randomized Trial of Vitamins C and E in the Prevention of Recurrence of Colorectal Polyps." *Cancer Research* 48 (1988): 4701–5.

Meyer, F., et al. "Interaction between Antioxidant Vitamin Supplementation and Cigarette Smoking during Radiation Therapy in Relation to Long-Term Effects on Recurrence and Mortality: A Randomized Trial among Head and Neck Cancer Patients." *International Journal of Cancer* 122 (2008): 1679–83.

Meyskens, F. J. "Role of Vitamin A and Its Derivatives in the Treatment of Human Cancer." In *Nutrients in Cancer Prevention and Treatment*, by K. N. Prasad and R. M. Williams, 349–263. Totawa, N.J.: Humana Press, 1995.

Meyskens, F. L. "Studies of Retinoids in the Prevention and Treatment of Cancer." *Journal of the American Academy of Dermatology* 6 (1982): 824–27.

Miller, E. R. III, et al. "Meta-Analysis: High-Dosage Vitamin E Supplementation May Increase All-Cause Mortality." *Annals of Internal Medicine* 142 (2005): 37–46.

Mills, E. E. "The Modifying Effect of Beta-carotene on Radiation and Chemotherapy Induced Oral Mucositis." *Br J Cancer* 57 (4) (1988): 416–17.

Misirlioglu, C. H., et al. "Pentoxifylline and Alpha-tocopherol in Prevention of Radiation-Induced Lung Toxicity in Patients with Lung Cancer." *Medical Oncology* 24 (2007): 308–11.

Miyajima, A., et al. "N-acetylcysteine Modifies Cis-dichlorodiammineplatinum-Induced Effects in Bladder Cancer Cells." *Japanese Journal of Cancer Research* 90 (1999): 565–70.

Morishige, F. "Studies on the Role of Large Dosage of Vitamin C in the Orthomolecular Nutritional Treatments of Cancer." Nakamura Memorial Hospital, Fukuoka, Japan, Ca 1983.

Murakami, C., et al. "Vitamin A-related Compounds, All-trans Retinal and Retinoic Acids, Selectively Inhibit Activities of Mammalian Replicative DNA Polymerases." *Biochimica et Biophysica Acta* 1574 (2002): 85–92.

Mutlu-Turkoglu, U., et al. "The Effect of Selenium and/or Vitamin E Treatments on Radiation-induced Intestinal Injury in Rats." *Life Sci* 66 (20) (2000): 1905–13.

Narra, V. R., et al. "Vitamins as Radioprotectors In Vivo. I. Protection by Vitamin C Against Internal Radionuclides in Mouse Testes: Implications to the Mechanism of Damage Caused by the Auger Effect." *Radiat Res* 137 (3) (1994): 394–99.

National Cancer Institute, Fact Sheet. "BRCA1 and BRCA2: Cancer Risk and Genetic Testing" (2009): 1–9.

Ni, Q. G., and Y. Pei. "Effect of Beta-carotene on 60Co-gamma-induced Mutation at T-lymphocyte Hypoxanthine-guanine Phosphoribosyl Transferase Locus in Rats." *Zhongguo Yao Li Xue Bao* 18 (6) (1997): 535–36.

Ntukidem, N. I., et al. "Estrogen Receptor genotypes, Menopausal Status, and the Lipid Effects of Tamoxifen." *Clin Pharmacol* 83 (2008): 702–10.

O'Connor, M. K., et al. "A Radioprotective Effect of Vitamin C Observed in Chinese Hamster Ovary Cells." *Br J Radiol* 50 (596) (1977): 587–91.

Okunieff, P., et al. "Antioxidants Reduce Consequences of Radiation Exposure." *Adv Exp Med Biol* 614 (2008): 165–78.

Okuno, M., et al. "Antiproliferative Effect of Carotenoids on Human Colon Cancer Cells without Conversion to Retinoic Acid." *Nutrition and Cancer* 32 (1998): 20–24.

Omenn, G. S., et.al. "Effects of a Combination of Beta-carotene and Vitamin A on Lung Cancer and Cardiovascular Disease." *New England Journal of Medicine* 334 (1996): 1150–55.

Pace, A., et al. "Neuroprotective Effect of Vitamin E Supplementation in Patients Treated with Cisplatin Chemotherapy." *Journal of Clinical Oncology* 21 (2003): 927–31.

Papova, L., et. al. "Micronucleus Test in Buccal Epithelium Cells from Patients Subjected to Paroramic Radiography." *Dentomaxillofac Radiol* 36 (2007): 168–71.

Pastorino, U., et al. "Adjuvant Treatment of Stage I Lung Cancer with High-Dose Vitamin A." *Journal of Clinical Oncology* 11 (1993): 1216–22.

Pathak, A. K., et al. "Chemotherapy Alone vs. Chemotherapy Plus High Dose Multiple Antioxidants in Patients with Advanced Non Small Cell Lung Cancer." *Journal of the American College of Nutrition* 24 (2005): 16–21.

Pierce, J. P., et al. "Influence of a Diet Very High in Vegetables, Fruit, and Fiber and Low in Fat on Prognosis Following Treatment for Breast Cancer: The Women's Healthy Eating and Living (WHEL) Randomized Trial. *JAMA* 298 (2007): 289–98.

Pollock, E. J., and G. J. Todaro. "Radiation Enhancement of SV40 Transformation in 3T3 and Human Cells." *Nature* 219 (5153) (1968): 520–21.

Prakash, P., N. I. Krinsky, and R. M. Russell. "Retinoids, Carotenoids, and Human Breast Cancer Cell Cultures: A Review of Differential Effects." *Nutrition Reviews* 58 (2000): 170–76.

Prasad, K. N. *Micronutrients in Health and Disease.* Boca Raton, Fla.: Taylor and Francis Group, 2011, pp. 1–365.

Prasad, K. N., W. Cole, and P. Hovland. "Cancer Prevention Studies: Past, Present, and Future Directions." *Nutrition* 14, no. 2 (1998): 197–210, 237–38.

Prasad, K. N., and J. Edwards-Prasad. "Effects of Tocopherol (vitamin E) Acid Succinate on Morphological Alterations and Growth Inhibition in Melanoma Cells in Culture." *Cancer Res* 42 (1982): 550–55.

———. "Vitamin E and Cancer Prevention: Recent Advances and Future Potentials." *Journal of the American College of Nutrition* 11 (1992): 487–500.

Prasad, K. N., and R. Kumar. "Effect of Individual and Multiple Antioxidant Vitamins on Growth and Morphology of Human Nontumorigenic and Tumorigenic Parotid Acinar Cells in Culture." *Nutrition and Cancer* 26 (1996): 11–19.

Prasad, K. N., et al. "Alpha-tocopheryl Succinate, the Most Effective Form of Vitamin E for Adjuvant Cancer Treatment: A Review." *J Am Coll Nutr* 22 (2) (2003): 108–17.

Prasad, K. N., et al. "Establishment and Characterization of Immortalized Cell Lines from Rat Parotid Glands." *In Vitro Cell Dev Biol Anim* 30A (5) (1994): 321–28.

Prasad, K. N., et al. "High Doses of Multiple Antioxidant Vitamins: Essential Ingredients in Improving the Efficacy of Standard Cancer Therapy." *Journal of the American College of Nutrition* 18 (1999): 13–25.

Prasad, K. N., et al. "Multiple Antioxidants in Prevention and Treatemnt of Alzheimer's

Disease: Analysis of Biological Rationale." *Clinical Neuropharmacology* 23 (2000): 2–13.

Prasad, K. N., et al. "Sodium Ascorbate Potentiates the Growth Inhibitory Effect of Certain Agents on Neuroblastoma Cells in Culture." *Proceedings of the National Academy of Science of the United States of America* 76 (1979): 829–32.

Prasad, K. N., W. C. Cole, and K. C. Prasad. "Risk Factors for Alzheimer's Disease: Role of Multiple Antioxidants, Non-steroidal Anti-inflammatory and Cholinergic Agents Alone or in Combination in Prevention and Treatment. *Journal of the American College of Nutrition.* 21 (2002): 506–22.

Prasad, K., L. Santamaria, and R. M. Williams. *Nutrients in Cancer Prevention and Treatment.* Totowa, N.J.: Humana Press, 1995.

Premkumar, V. G., et al. "Anti-angiogenic Potential of Coenzyme Q10, Riboflavin and Niacin in Breast Cancer Patients Undergoing Tamoxifen Therapy." *Vascular Pharmacology* 48 (2008): 191–201.

Pryor, W. A., "Oxidants and Antioxidants." *Natural Antioxidants in Human Health and Disease*, by B. Frei, 1–24. New York: Academy Press, Inc., 1994.

Puck, T. T., et al. "Caffeine Enhanced Measurement of Mutagenesis by Low Levels of Gamma-irradiation in Human Lymphocytes." *Somat Cell Mol Genet* 19 (5) (1993): 423–29.

Pukkala, E., A. Auvinen, and G. Wahlberg. "Incidence of Cancer Among Finnish Airline Cabin Attendants, 1967–92." *BMJ* 311 (7006) (1995): 649–52.

Qiao, Y. L., et al. "Total and Cancer Mortality after Supplementation with Vitamins and Minerals: Follow-up of the Linxian General Population Nutrition Intervention Trial." *Journal of the National Cancer Institute* 101 (2009): 507–18.

Radner, B. S. , and A. R. Kennedy. "Suppression of X-ray Induced Transformation by Vitamin E in Mouse C3H/10T1/2 Cells." *Cancer Lett* 32 (1) (1986): 25–32.

Rafnsson, V., et al. "Risk of Breast Cancer in Female Flight Attendants: A Population-based Study (Iceland)." *Cancer Causes Control* 12 (2) (2001): 95–101.

Ramakrishnan, N., W. W. Wolfe, and G. N. Catravas. "Radioprotection of Hematopoietic Tissues in Mice by Lipoic Acid." *Radiat Res* 130 (3) (1992): 360–65.

Rao, C. V., and B. S. Reddy. "Modulating Effect and Type of Dietary Fat on Ornithine Decarboxylase Tyrosine Protein Kinase and Prostaglandins Production During Colon Carcinogenesis." *Carcinogenesis* 14 (1993): 1327.

Reddy B. S., C. Sharma, and E. Wynder. "Fecal Factors Which Modify the Formation of Fecal Co-mutagens in High and Low-risk Population for Colon Cancer." *Cancer Lett* 10 (1980): 123–32.

Reddy, B. S. "Dietary Fat, Calories, and Fiber in Colon Cancer." *Prev Med* 22 (1993): 738.

Reliene, R., and R. H. Schiestl. "Antioxidant N-acetylcysteine Reduces Incidence and Multiplicity of Lymphoma in Atm Deficient Mice." *DNA Repair* 5 (2006): 852–59.

Reznick, A. Z., et al. "Modification of Plasma Proteins by Cigarette Smoke as Measured by Protein Carbonyl Formation." *Biochemical Journal* 286 (1992): 607–11.

Rice, H. E., et al. "Review of Radiation Risks from Computed Tomography: Essentials for the Pediatric Surgeon." *J Pediatr Surg* 42 (4) (2007): 603–7.

Richardson, M. A., et al. "Complementary/Alternative Medicine Use in a Comprehensive Cancer Center and the Implications for Oncology." *Journal of Clinical Oncology* 18 (2000): 2505–14.

Robbins, E. "Radiation Risks from Imaging Studies in Children with Cancer." *Pediatr Blood Cancer* 51 (4) (2008): 453–57.

Rodrigues, M. J., A. Bouyon, and J. Alexandre. "Role of Antioxidant Complements and Supplements in Oncology in Addition to an Equilibrate Regimen: A Systematic Review." *Bull Cancer* 96 (2009): 677–84.

Roffe, L., K. Schmidt, and E. Ernst. "Efficacy of Coenzyme Q10 for Improved Tolerability of Cancer Treatments: A Systematic Review." *Journal of Clinical Oncology* 22 (2004): 4418–24.

Roncucci, L., et al. "Antioxidant Vitamins or Lactulose for the Prevention of the Recurrence of Colorectal Adenomas. Colorectal Cancer Study Group of the University of Modena and the Health Care District 16." *Diseases of the Colon and Rectum* 36 (1993): 227–34.

Rossi, C., et al. "Intestinal Tumour Chemoprevention with the Antioxidant Lipoic Acid Stimulates the Growth of Breast Cancer." *European Journal of Cancer* 44 (2008): 2696–704.

Rothkamm, K., and M. Lobrich. "Evidence for a Lack of DNA Double-strand Break Repair in Human Cells Exposed to Very Low X-ray Doses." *Proc Natl Acad Sci U S A* 100 (9) (2003): 5057–62.

Rusciani, L., et al. "Recombinant Interferon Alpha-2b and Coenzyme Q10 as a Postsurgical Adjuvant Therapy for Melanoma: A 3-Year Trial with Recombinant Interferon-alpha and 5-Year Follow-Up." *Melanoma Research* 17 (2007): 177–83.

Sachdanandam, P. "Antiangiogenic and Hypolipidemic Activity of Coenzyme Q10 Supplementation to Breast Cancer Patients Undergoing Tamoxifen Therapy." *Biofactors* 32 (2008): 151–59.

Sakano, K., et al. "Suppression of Azoxymethane-Induced Colonic Premalignant Lesion Formation by Coenzyme Q10 in Rats." *Asian Pacific Journal of Cancer Prevention* 7 (2006): 599–603.

Salganik, R. I. "The Benefits and Hazards of Antioxidants: Controlling Apoptosis and Other Protective Mechanisms in Cancer Patients and the Human Population." *Journal of the American College of Nutrition* 20 (2001): 464S–472S, discussion 473S–475S.

Santamaria, L., A. Bianchi, and G. Mobilio. "Cancer Prevention by Carotenoids." In *Nutrition, Growth and Cancer*, edited by G. P. Tryfiates and K. N. Prasad, 177. Alan R. Liss, Inc.: New York, 1988.

Satia, J. A., et al. "Long-Term Use of Beta-carotene, Retinol, Lycopene, and Lutein Supplements and Lung Cancer Risk: Results from the VITamins And Lifestyle (VITAL) Study." *American Journal of Epidemiology* 169 (2009): 815–28.

Sato, R., et al. "Prospective Study of Carotenoids, Tocopherols, and Retinoid Concentrations and the Risk of Breast Cancer." *Cancer Epidemiology, Biomarkers and Prevention* 11 (2002): 451–57.

Schatzkin, A., et al. "Lack of Effect of a Low-Fat, High-Fiber Diet on the Recurrence of Colorectal Adenomas. Polyp Prevention Trial Study Group." *New England Journal of Medicine* 342 (2000): 1149–55.

Schectman, G., J. C. Byrd, and R. Hoffmann. "Ascorbic Acid Requirements for Smokers: Analysis of a Population Survey." *American Journal of Clinical Nutrition* 53 (1991): 1466–70.

Seifried, H. E., et al. "The Antioxidant Conundrum in Cancer." *Cancer Research* 63 (2003): 4295–98.

Seifter, E., et al. "Vitamin A and Beta-carotene as Adjunctive Therapy to Tumor Excision, Radiation Therapy and Chemotherapy." In *Vitamins, Nutrition and Cancer*. Basel: Karger, 1984.

Shah, N. B., and S. L. Platt. "ALARA: Is There a Cause for Alarm? Reducing Radiation Risks from Computed Tomography Scanning in Children." *Curr Opin Pediatr* 20 (3) (2008): 243–47.

Shike, M., et al. "Lack of Effect of a Low-Fat, High-Fruit, -Vegetable, and -Fiber Diet on Serum Prostate-Specific Antigen of Men without Prostate Cancer: Results from a Randomized Trial." *Journal of Clinical Oncology* 20 (2002): 3592–98.

Shults, C. W., et al. "Effects of Coenzyme Q10 in Early Parkinson's Disease: Evidence of Slowing of the Functional Decline." *Archives of Neurology* 59 (2002): 1541–50.

Sigurdson, A. J., and E. Ron. "Cosmic Radiation Exposure and Cancer Risk Among Flight Crew." *Cancer Invest* 22 (5) (2004): 743–61.

Simeone, A. M., and A. M. Tari. "How Retinoids Regulate Breast Cancer Cell Proliferation and Apoptosis." *Cellular and Molecular Life Sciences* 61 (2005): 1475–84.

Song, Y. J., et al. "Coffee, Tea, Colas, and Risk of Epithelial Ovarian Cancer." *Cancer Epidemiol Biomarkers Prev* 17 (3) (2008): 712–16.

Steck-Scott, S., et al. "Carotenoids, Vitamin A and Risk of Adenomatous Polyp Recurrence in the Polyp Prevention Trial." *International Journal of Cancer* 112 (2004): 295–305.

Stich, H. F., et al. "Remission of Oral Leukoplakias and Micronuclei in Tobacco/Betel Quid Chewers Treated with Beta-carotene and with Beta-carotene Plus Vitamin A." *International Journal of Cancer* 42 (1988): 195–99.

Stich, H. F., et al. "Remission of Oral Precancerous Lesions of Tobacco/Arecanut Chewers Following Administration of Beta-carotene or Vitamin A, and Maintenance of the Protective Effect." *Cancer Detection and Prevention* 15 (1991): 93–98.

Stolzenberg-Solomon, R. Z., et al. "Vitamin E Intake, Alpha-tocopherol Status, and Pancreatic Cancer in a Cohort of Male Smokers." *American Journal of Clinical Nutrition* 89 (2009): 584–91.

Sun, Y. X., et al. "Mechanism of Ascorbic Acid-Induced Reversion against Malignant

Phenotype in Human Gastric Cancer Cells." *Biomedical and Environmental Sciences* 19 (2006): 385–91.

Suzuki, K., S. Kodama, and M. Watanabe. "Extremely Low-dose Ionizing Radiation Causes Activation of Mitogen-activated Protein Kinase Pathway and Enhances Proliferation of Normal Human Diploid Cells." *Cancer Res* 61 (14) (2001): 5396–401.

Szostek, S., et al. "Herpes Viruses as Possible Cofactors in HPV-16-Related Oncogenesis." *Acta Biochim Pol* (2009).

Tamimi, R. M., et al. "Plasma Carotenoids, Retinol, and Tocopherols and Risk of Breast Cancer." *American Journal of Epidemiology* 161 (2005): 153–60.

Tang, N. P., et al. "Flavonoids Intake and Risk of Lung Cancer: A Meta-Analysis." *Japanese Journal of Clinical Oncology* 39 (2009): 352–59.

Tavani, A., et al. "Coffee and Alcohol Intake and Risk of Ovarian Cancer: An Italian Case-Control Study." *Nutr Cancer* 39 (1) (2001): 29–34.

Theis, R. P., et al. "Smoking, Environmental Tobacco Smoke, and Risk of Renal Cell Cancer: A Population-based Case-control Study." *BMC Cancer* 8 (2008): 387.

Thibault, A., et al. "Phase I Study of Phenylacetate Administered Twice Daily to Patients with Cancer." *Cancer* 75 (2009): 2932.

Thiebaut, A. C., et al. "Dietary Intakes of Omega-6 and Omega-3 Polyunsaturated Fatty Acids and the Risk of Breast Cancer." *International Journal of Cancer* 124 (2009): 924–31.

Thomson, C. A., et al. "The Role of Antioxidants and Vitamin A in Ovarian Cancer: Results from the Women's Health Initiative." *Nutrition and Cancer* 60 (2008): 710–19.

Tillmann, T., et al. "Carcinogenicity Study of GSM and DCS Wireless Communication Signals in B6C3F1 Mice." *Bioelectromagnetics* 28 (3) (2007): 173–87.

Toth, B., and K. Patil. "Enhancing Effect of Vitamin E on Murine Intestinal Tumorigenesis by 1,2-dimethylhydrazine Dihydrochloride." *Journal of the National Cancer Institute* 70 (1983): 1107–11.

Tworoger, S. S., et al. "Caffeine, Alcohol, Smoking, and the Risk of Incident Epithelial Ovarian Cancer." *Cancer* 112 (5) (2008): 1169–77.

Umegaki, K., et al. "Feeding Mice Palm Carotene Prevents DNA Damage in Bone Marrow and Reduction of Peripheral Leukocyte Counts, and Enhances Survival Following X-ray Irradiation." *Carcinogenesis* 18 (10) (1997): 1943–47.

Ushakova, T., et al. "Modification of Gene Expression by Dietary Antioxidants in Radiation-induced Apoptosis of Mice Splenocytes." *Free Radic Biol Med* 26 (7–8) (1999): 887–91.

van Breemen, R. B., and N. Pajkovic. "Multitargeted Therapy of Cancer by Lycopene." *Cancer Letters* 269 (2008): 339–51.

van Zandwijk, et al. "EUROSCAN, a Randomized Trial of Vitamin A and N-acetylcysteine in Patients with Head and Neck Cancer or Lung Cancer. For the European Organization for Research and Treatment of Head and Neck and Lung Cancer Cooperative Groups." *Journal of the National Cancer Institute* 92 (2000): 977–86.

Venkateswaran, V., et al. "A Combination of Micronutrients Is Beneficial in Reducing the Incidence of Prostate Cancer and Increasing Survival in the Lady Transgenic Model." *Cancer Prevention Research* 2 (2009): 473–83.

Venugopal, D., et al. "Reduction of Estrogen-Induced Transformation of Mouse Mammary Epithelial Cells by N-acetylcysteine." *Journal of Steroid Biochemistry and Molecular Biology* 109 (2008): 22–30.

Verma, A., et al. "Selenomethionine Stimulates MAPK (ERK) Phosphorylation, Protein Oxidation, and DNA Synthesis in Gastric Cancer Cells." *Nutrition and Cancer* 49 (2004): 184–90.

Verrax, J., and P. B. Calderon. "Pharmacologic Concentrations of Ascorbate Are Achieved by Parenteral Administration and Exhibit Antitumoral Effects." *Free Radical Biology and Medicine* 47 (2009): 32–40.

Vogel, V. G., et al. "Update of the National Surgical Adjuvant Breast and Bowel Project Study of Tamoxifen and Raloxifene (STAR) P-2 Trial: Preventing Breast Cancer." *Cancer Prev. Res (phila)* 3(6) (2010): 646–706.

Wactawski-Wende, J., et.al. "Calcium Plus Vitamin D Supplementation and the Risk of Colorectal Cancer." *N Engl J Med* 354 (7) (2006): 684–96.

Walker, E. M., et al. "Nutritional and High Dose Antioxidant Interventions During Radiation Therapy for Cancer of the Breast." Presented at International Conference on Nutrition and Cancer, Montevideo, Uruguay, July, 2002.

Walser, T., et al. "Smoking and Lung Cancer: The Role of Inflammation." *Proc Am Thorac Soc* 5 (8) (2008): 811–15.

Wan, M. J., et al. "Acute Appendicitis in Young Children: Cost-effectiveness of US Versus CT in Diagnosis—A Markov Decision Analytic Model." *Radiology*, 2008.

Wan, X. S., et al. "Protection Against Radiation-induced Oxidative Stress in Cultured Human Epithelial Cells by Treatment with Antioxidant Agents." *Int J Radiat Oncol Biol Phys* 64 (5) (2006): 1475–81.

Wang, L., et al. "Dietary Intake of Selected Flavonols, Flavones, and Flavonoid-rich Foods and Risk of Cancer in Middle-Aged and Older Women." *American Journal of Clinical Nutrition* 89 (2009): 905–12.

Wang, Y. J., M. C. Yang, and M. H. Pan. "Dihydrolipoic Acid Inhibits Tetrachlorohydroquinone-Induced Tumor Promotion through Prevention of Oxidative Damage." *Food and Chemical Toxicology* 46 (2008): 3739–48.

Weinberg, R. B., et al. "Pro-oxidant Effect of Vitamin E in Cigarette Smokers Consuming a High Polyunsaturated Fat Diet." *Arteriosclerosis, Thrombosis, and Vascular Biology* 21 (2001): 1029–33.

Weingarten, M. A., A. Zalmanovici, and J. Yaphe. "Dietary Calcium Supplementation for Preventing Colorectal Cancer and Adenomatous Polyps." *Cochrane Database of Systematic Reviews* (2008): CD003548.

Weinstein, S. J., et al. "Serum Alpha-tocopherol and Gamma-tocopherol in Relation to Prostate Cancer Risk in a Prospective Study." *Journal of the National Cancer Institute* 97 (2005): 396–99.

Weinstein, S. J., et al. "Serum and Dietary Vitamin E in Relation to Prostate Cancer Risk." *Cancer Epidemiology, Biomarkers and Prevention* 16 (2007): 1253–59.

Weiss, J. F., and M. R. Landauer. "Protection Against Ionizing Rradiation by Antioxidant Nutrients and Phytochemicals." *Toxicology* 189 (1–2) (2003): 1–20.

———. "Radioprotection by Antioxidants." *Ann N Y Acad Sci* 899 (2000): 44–60.

Williams, A. W., et al. "Beta-carotene Modulates Human Prostate Cancer Cell Growth and May Undergo Intracellular Metabolism to Retinol." *Journal of Nutrition* 130 (2000): 728–32.

Witenberg, B., et al. "Ascorbic Acid Inhibits Apoptosis Induced by X Irradiation in HL60 Myeloid Leukemia Cells." *Radiation Research* 152 (1999): 468–78.

Wogan, G. N., et al. "Environmental and Chemical Carcinogenesis." *Semin Cancer Biol* 14 (6) (2004): 473–86.

Wybieralska, E., et al. "Ascorbic Acid Inhibits the Migration of Walker 256 Carcinosarcoma Cells." *Cellular and Molecular Biology Letters* 13 (2008): 103–11.

Wynder, E. L., F. R. Lemon, and I. J. Bross. "Cancer and Coronary Artery Disease Among Seventh-day Adventists." *Cancer* (12) (1959): 1016–28. Yang, Q., et al. "Serum Folate and Cancer Mortality among U.S. Adults: Findings from the Third National Health and Nutritional Examination Survey Linked Mortality File." *Cancer Epidemiology, Biomarkers and Prevention* 18 (2009): 1439–47.

Yusuf, S., et al. "Vitamin E Supplementation and Cardiovascular Events in High-Risk Patients. The Heart Outcomes Prevention Evaluation Study Investigators." *New England Journal of Medicine* 342 (2000): 154–60.

Yuvaraj, S., et al. "Ameliorating Effect of Coenzyme Q10, Riboflavin and Niacin in Tamoxifen-Treated Postmenopausal Breast Cancer Patients with Special Reference to Lipids and Lipoproteins." *Clinical Biochemistry* 40 (2007): 623–28.

Zhang, S. M. "Role of Vitamins in the Risk, Prevention, and Treatment of Breast Cancer." *Current Opinion in Obstetrics and Gynecology* 16 (2004): 19–25.

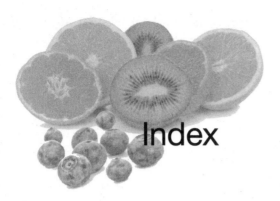

Index

Page numbers in *italics* refer to tables.

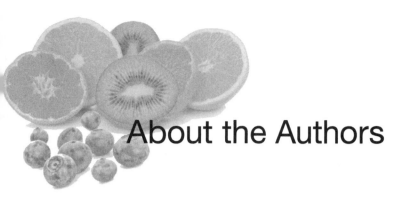

About the Authors

KEDAR N. PRASAD, PH.D.

Kedar N. Prasad obtained a master's degree in zoology from the University of Bihar, Ranchi, India, and a Ph.D. in radiation biology from the University of Iowa, Iowa City, in 1963. He received postdoctoral training at the Brookhaven National Laboratory, Long Island, New York, and joined the Department of Radiology at the University of Colorado Health Sciences Center, where he became professor and director for the Center for Vitamins and Cancer Research. He has published more than two hundred articles in peer-reviewed journals and authored and edited fifteen books on radiation biology, nutrition and cancer, and nutrition and neurological diseases, particularly Alzheimer's disease and Parkinson's disease. These articles were published in highly prestigious journals such as *Science, Nature,* and *Proceedings of the National Academy of Sciences of the United States of America.* Dr. Prasad has received many honors, including the invitation by the Nobel Prize Committee to nominate a candidate for the Nobel Prize in medicine for 1982; the 1999 Harold Harper Lecture at the meeting of the American College of Advancement in Medicine; an award for the best review of 1998–1999 on antioxidants and cancer and 1999–2000 on antioxidants and Parkinson's disease by the American College of Nutrition. He is a Fellow of the American College of Nutrition and served as president of the International Society of Nutrition and Cancer from 1992–2000. He belongs to several professional societies, such as the American Association for Cancer Research and the Radiation Research Society. Currently he is chief scientific officer of the Premier Micronutrient Corporation.

K. CHE PRASAD, M.S., M.D.

K. Che Prasad, M.S., M.D., received his bachelor's degree with highest honors in human integrative biology from the University of California—Berkeley. He was elected to Phi Beta Kappa as a junior and made an original discovery that alpha-tocopheryl succinate (vitamin E) enhances the effects of naturally occurring substances, such as adenosine 3',5'-cyclic monophosphate (cAMP), on growth inhibition and differentiation in melanoma cells. After receiving his undergraduate degree in 1991, he entered the University of California—Berkeley/University of California—San Francisco Joint Medical Program, from which he received a master's degree in health and medical sciences in 1995 and an M.D. in 1997. Dr. K. Che Prasad completed his residency in anatomic and clinical Pathology, including a fellowship in surgical pathology, at the University of California—San Francisco in 2002. He is currently working as a pathologist with Marin Medical Laboratories, where he is director of microbiology and codirector of cytology. He is a member of the College of American Pathologists, the California Society of Pathologists, and the Marin Medical Society.